"Does anyone understand how we feel?"

You've suffered the heartache of infertility. The trying and wondering. The hope and the disappointment.

Alan and Patricia Trent have walked the same path. Felt the same hurt and frustration.

They understand.

From their personal experience, and from their research into the options infertile couples face, the Trents have prepared this compassionate, practical book.

Barren Couples, Broken Hearts

. . . will encourage you. Give you help and hope.

Best of all, it introduces you to a man and woman who *do* understand exactly how you feel— and who care enough to help.

BARREN
Couples

♥ ♥ ♥

BROKEN
Hearts

Alan Trent &
Patricia Hatfield Trent

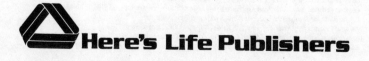
Here's Life Publishers

First Printing, October 1991

Published by
HERE'S LIFE PUBLISHERS, INC.
P. O. Box 1576
San Bernardino, CA 92402

Library of Congress Cataloging-in-Publication Data
Trent, Alan.
    Barren couples, broken hearts : a compassionate look at
infertility / Alan and Patricia Trent.
      p.   cm.
    ISBN 0-89840-325-1
    1. Infertility. 2. Infertility–Religious aspects–Christianity.
I. Trent, Patricia. II. Title.
RC889.T74   1991
616.6'92–dc20   91-4948
                             CIP

Scripture quotations are from the *Good News Bible: The Bible in Today's English Version*, © 1966, 1971, 1976 by the American Bible Society.

Cover design by Michelle Treiber

For More Information, Write:
L.I.F.E.–P.O. Box A399, Sydney South 2000, Australia
Campus Crusade for Christ of Canada–Box 300, Vancouver, B.C., V6C 2X3, Canada
Campus Crusade for Christ–Pearl Assurance House, 4 Temple Row, Birmingham, B2 5HG, England
Lay Institute for Evangelism–P.O. Box 8786, Auckland 3, New Zealand
Campus Crusade for Christ–P.O. Box 240, Raffles City Post Office, Singapore 9117
Great Commission Movement of Nigeria–P.O. Box 500, Jos, Plateau State Nigeria, West Africa
Campus Crusade for Christ International–Arrowhead Springs, San Bernardino, CA 92414, U.S.A.

Contents

Foreword

Barren Couples, Broken Hearts by Alan and Patricia Trent deals with infertility, an increasingly prevalent difficulty of couples in their childbearing years. Infertility was a pressing concern of several couples whose stories are recorded in the Bible. For example, Abraham and Sarah were childless into their very advanced years. God visited them and assured them He would fulfill His promise that they would become parents of a nation of people. Isaac was born unto them and that new nation was begun. Hannah poured out her complaint to God that she was barren; God heard her prayer and she gave birth to Samuel. The parents of Samson were without children and God's messengers visited them, assuring them they would have a child.

In the New Testament, Zechariah and Elizabeth, the parents of John the Baptist, were advanced in years before they were blessed by the birth of a son. These stories bear witness: God intends that couples who desire children should have them. In this sense, this book is a prophetic witness of God in their quest to become parents.

The process of conception, gestation, and birth of children is one of the most mysterious events in human life. The medical profession has amassed an elaborate array of options, yet it is outwitted when a couple has tried all the technology to no avail. Often, the couple then adopts a child and shortly thereafter the wife becomes pregnant! We are aided tremendously by medical wisdom and technology, but possibly the act of surrender itself has some spiritual-biological mystery that needs exploration.

The Trents have expended tremendous effort and discipline in the creation of this book. They have thoroughly researched the options for parenthood and have presented the material in an exceptionally readable manner. They take a highly emotional issue, that of an unfulfilled desire for children, and treat it in a gentle and wise way without gushing with frothy sentimentality.

If you are a pastor you will find this book to be a marvelous aid as you deal with infertile couples, and one you can readily recommend. If you are a person suffering from the frustration and anxiety of childlessness, you hold a compassionate and wise guidebook for your pilgrimage toward parenthood. If you are a yearning parent of a childless young couple, this book will enhance your empathy and temper your expectations, making you wiser and kinder in your eagerness to become a grandparent. If you are a seminary professor of pastoral care, this book can be excellent parallel reading for classes in which you discuss parenthood. You may find, as I have, that students themselves sometimes struggle with the problem of infertility.

The audience for the message of the Trents is wide and varied. The authors have tapped a profound, private grief that many people bear which is often the subject of crass humor and aggressive teasing. As you read this book, you will be tutored in empathy and kindness toward those who yearn for children.

WAYNE E. OATES, PH.D.
Professor of Psychiatry and Behavioral Sciences
University of Louisville School of Medicine
Senior Professor of Psychology of Religion
The Southern Baptist Theological Seminary
Louisville, Kentucky

Having children is natural, something that comes almost automatically with marriage. That, we understood, was the law of the universe.

1
When the Promise Is Broken

Alan

IT WAS Sunday morning, a day when years of frustration, pain, emotional and spiritual struggle were coming to an end and a new life was beginning. Just a few weeks before, Patricia and I had adopted a baby girl. This was the day we had chosen for our dedication as new parents.

Since I was pastor of our church, I had asked the professor who was supervising my doctoral work to preach that morning's dedication sermon. Another colleague, a chaplain at a local college, would handle the litany of commitment.

As parishioners began arriving I went into the sanctuary to make sure everything was ready. While talking with friends, I noticed a young woman come in and sit in her usual place in the pew. She took off her coat and opened the church bulletin. Suddenly her expression changed and she looked as if she were about to break into tears. Quietly she stood up, put on her coat, and walked with head bowed toward the rear doors.

I wasn't sure what was wrong, but I had a pretty good idea. I didn't know her and her husband well, but I knew they had no children. One of the good things about being a minister is that people expect you to speak to them when it looks as if something might be wrong. Deciding to use my pastoral prerogative, I excused myself from the conversation and cut down a back hallway where I knew I could intercept this lady before she left the church.

"Are you okay?" I asked.

"Well, not really. It's just me. I can't stay today. It's not the church or anything, just me," she said, not daring to look up.

"Is it the baby dedication?" I asked.

"Please don't misunderstand," she said, as the tears began to come. "I really am happy for you two. I know you've wanted a baby for a long time. But I just can't stay. It hurts too much."

At that moment all I could say was that I understood, and that I would be in touch. We'd set up a time when she and her husband and I could get together and talk about it.

I understood very well. For the better part of the last six years I'd watched helplessly, sometimes filled with despair, sometimes raging in anger, as I saw the same pained expression on my wife's face. I remembered similar Sundays when she hurt too much to sit through the many dedication services I was asked to lead. I understood something of what this young woman and her husband must be feeling— the hopelessness, the hurt, the sense of being cheated. And the more I've learned about infertility over these last few years, through both personal experience and research, the more I'm convinced this same scene is played out somewhere almost every Sunday morning.

Infertile couples differ a great deal from those who have no problem having children. During holidays, when everyone else is enjoying the spirit of the season, we may find ourselves plunged into a deep depression that can last for weeks. Sometimes we feel like outcasts, even in our own worship community. All of its emphasis on "family night" and other family-oriented programs serves to remind us that we don't fit in. We've been taught that a "real family" is a mom, a dad, two children, a dog, and a cat living in a house in the suburbs.

We are constantly reminded of what we do not have. Shopping malls are full of children and pregnant women. We feel the ache inside when we pass the baby food section at the supermarket. An invitation to a baby shower can trigger a two-hour crying spell.

We are men and women who feel acutely the betrayal of a broken promise. This wasn't supposed to happen—at least not to us. Having children is natural, something that comes almost automatically with marriage. That, we understood, was the law of the universe, as deeply ingrained in the created order as sunrise and sunset. But for us it wasn't happening.

Worse, there came a time when our deepest fears told us it might never happen. So we felt betrayed, not just by nature, but by God Himself. After all, didn't He say to the first couple, "Be fruitful and multiply, fill the earth and subdue it" (Genesis 1:28)?

This book is about coping, about understanding the landslide of emotions and how they affect us and our marriage. It's about our intense spiritual struggle. Make no mistake, infertility is a very real spiritual struggle. Our faith is thrown into chaos. The beliefs that once sustained us, our trust in a loving and caring God, are shattered like crystal on the harsh anvil of reality. Not a few couples lose their faith as they wander through an emotional wilderness where nothing in life seems certain any more.

But this is also a book about finding that faith again, and about alternatives—what we can do when natural conception is no longer an option. These alternatives, however, demand that we examine our personal beliefs very closely so that we will choose wisely. Choosing carelessly can bring as much pain as childlessness.

If we are to understand what is happening to us, we must begin with a brief look at our malady. While the following discussion is by no means exhaustive, it may help us realize the complexity of our situation.

What Is Infertility?

Having a baby should be so simple. The basic necessities for conception are ovulation, healthy fallopian tubes, and good quality sperm. At first glance the process appears elementary. An egg is released from the ovary and travels into the fallopian tube. Sperm enter the vagina and swim through the uterus up into the fallopian tube where one of them fertilizes the egg. Moving through the fallopian tube into the uterus, the fertilized egg, now a small cluster of cells, attaches itself to the endometrium where it develops into a fetus.

It sounds so simple, but in reality it isn't. Any number of things may go wrong along the way.

Infertility is a physical disease in which the male and/or female body's natural capacity for reproduction is impaired. An infertile man or woman is one who has less than the maximum potential for conception. For the most part it is a temporary condition, not to be confused with sterility, which is permanent. It is a disease that affects every aspect of our lives: our bodies, our minds, our emotions, our spiritual lives, and our relationships with spouse and family.

Doctors define infertility as the inability to conceive after six months of regular intercourse without contraception. Roughly 15 percent of the married couples in the United States have fertility problems. That's about 3.5 million people, or about one couple out of every six.[1]

Causes of Infertility

Infertility may have any number of causes. As Robert H. Blank, an infertility specialist, points out, the sperm count of American males has fallen 30 percent over the last half century. He estimates that as many as 25 percent of American males have sperm counts low enough for them to be considered sterile.[2]

Contemporary lifestyles play an important role in the infertility epidemic. Many couples put off trying to start a family until both husband and wife are well established in their careers. This often means waiting until their late twenties or even early thirties before attempting conception. By then reproductive capacity in both male and female has already begun to decline, simply because of age. Thus the longer a couple waits to get started, the greater the likelihood of a problem developing, and the fewer years they have left to discover and attempt to correct it.

We also may be reaping some of the more negative benefits of the sexual revolution. Blank writes:

> Contemporary social patterns, including increased sexual contact of young women with a variety of partners, appear to be linked with increased infertility in women. The epidemic proportions of gonorrhea and more recently of herpes simplex II among young women promises to accentuate this problem.[3]

Stress also may be a culprit. While most researchers agree that stress does not cause infertility, they do point out that stress may exacerbate already existing difficulties. High levels of stress, for example, may interfere with ovulation.[4]

This doesn't mean all those well-meaning folks who offer cheap advice—"Just relax; then you'll get pregnant"—are right. They aren't. The cause of infertility is very much in the body and not in the mind. What it does mean is that stress is simply one more factor that can make things worse, physically as well as emotionally.

A host of other influences may decrease our chances of having a child. Pesticides, exposure to radiation, and toxins encountered in the workplace, such as industrial solvents, have been found to damage sperm. Abuse of so-called recreational drugs such as marijuana, cocaine, LSD, alcohol, and tobacco also may have detrimental effects. Certain birth control methods, such as the IUD, are known to increase fertility problems by causing pelvic infections. And the pill, in such wide use today, may contribute to some cases by causing faulty ovulation or by interfering with a woman's natural hormonal balance.

Physical impairments may reduce reproductive capacity. Among males, low sperm count is a primary factor. Sperm may have "low motility," which means they are unable to swim through the female body far enough to reach the egg. Low penetration is another problem, in which sperm are simply too weak to make it through the woman's cervical mucus. Autoimmunity, a condition that causes sperm to be immobilized by the male's own antibodies, also reduces sperm production. Sexually transmitted diseases such as gonorrhea may obstruct the canals through which sperm must travel. Many males suffer from varicocele, or varicose veins in the testes. This causes the temperature in the scrotum to rise, killing some of the sperm. Various systemic disorders, such as diabetes, may have an adverse effect. And finally, there may be some form of sexual dysfunction, such as premature ejaculation.

The female reproductive system is even more susceptible to malfunction. There may be difficulties with ovulation. Researchers estimate that half of all female infertility is related to problems with the ovaries and release of eggs. Pelvic Inflammatory Disease (PID), endometriosis, or bacterial infections of the cervical area may prohibit the sperm from uniting with the egg. Hyperprolactinemia, a condition where high levels of the hormone prolactin are released into the bloodstream, may cause irregular menstrual periods.[5]

Getting pregnant should be so simple, but it isn't. These are only a handful of the myriad things that may at any time, through no fault of our own, go wrong with our reproductive systems. Physicians estimate that roughly 40 percent of the time the difficulty is found in the male, 40 percent of the time in the female, and 20 percent of the time a combination of both.[6]

Hope Through New Technologies

Though the difficulties may seem insurmountable, there is hope. The infertility epidemic has given rise to an entirely new medical phenomenon: alternative reproductive technology. As a result, many previously unheard of options are available to the childless couple, above and beyond the frequently chosen alternative of adoption. New surgical techniques make it possible to repair damaged fallopian tubes and varicocele. Developments in drug therapy may increase ovulation or regulate the menstrual cycle. And there is the brave new world of fertility clinics, where artificial insemination, *in vitro* fertilization, artificial embryonation, and embryo adoption may be offered to clients who are incapable of natural conception. Surrogate motherhood—currently much disputed in the courts—is even considered by the few couples who dare brave the legal and emotional minefields.

Personal Struggles

Infertility is, however, a disease that affects much more than the body. It impacts our self-esteem, how we think of ourselves as male or female, husband or wife. Our marriage, and our relationships with family and friends, may be plunged into chaos as we struggle to accomplish what comes naturally for so many others. It can leave us feeling trapped in an emotional maze of depression and other negative feelings. And our religious life, so often a comfort in other crises, may itself become an intimate part of our struggle.

I had been in my first pastorate just over a year when our struggle, which was to last over six years, began. Patricia and I began to suspect something was wrong when she was unable to get pregnant after being off birth control for a year. On our first visit to the doctor, who wasn't an infertility specialist, he sent me for a sperm test and Patricia for an exam to see whether her fallopian tubes were open. Both tests came back positive. The doctor said there was nothing wrong, that we probably just hadn't "gotten lucky" yet. "Just be patient," he said. "Keep taking your basal temperature and be sure to have sex at your most fertile times of the cycle. If you aren't pregnant in a year, then come back to see me."

Patricia

During that year Alan and I were increasingly busy. He had just started his doctoral work and I was studying for the C.P.A. exam. I did all the right things, took my temperature, recorded the highs and lows on the chart the doctor had given me. Still the months went by and nothing happened. It was then that I began to think something serious might be wrong with me. It had to be me, since Alan's test result was normal.

I'd had a bad case of appendicitis when I was in elementary school, and I remember the doctor telling my mother that when I grew up I might need to see a doctor about my having a baby. Of course that meant nothing to me then. But now, as the months went by I began to think, "What if I can't get pregnant? What if I can *never* have a baby?"

It seemed that no matter how hard I worked at my new job, studied, or prayed, that terrible thought always lurked in the back of my mind. I had always suffered from tension headaches, but now they were worse. There were several young couples in our church, all with new babies or young children. Whenever someone had a new baby a rose was placed on the altar. And every time I saw that, my stomach hurt. It was a reminder telling me again and again that I couldn't do what all these other women could.

Eventually it got so bad that I couldn't bring myself to go to church those Sundays after there had been a new arrival in somebody's family. No one said anything. For the most part these were very loving, supportive people. But every time I went through those doors it seemed like I had a sign around my neck that read "defective" or something. The mothers would talk about their babies and kids. It was easy to see that their children were the most important things in their lives. All I could talk about was tax law and audits. I never felt more alone, more left out, in my entire life. My church and my faith had gotten me through many crises before, but now they only added to the pain and depression that hovered like a black cloud over my every day.

Conclusion

These are the subjects that will occupy the greater part of our discussion in the chapters ahead. To deal successfully with this crisis, we must address the whole person—body, mind, and spirit—along with our marriage. We must learn how to bring healing to our emotions and to our spiritual life. We must struggle with our faith, daring to wrestle with God, believing that if we search diligently for answers, they will come. And we cannot avoid grappling with the moral and ethical questions surrounding some of the reproductive techniques now available to childless couples.

THINGS TO DO

1. If you have not gotten pregnant after six months without birth control, you both need to see your doctor. The sooner you begin, the better your chances.

2. Talk openly with each other. Negative feelings and emotional pain such as depression and feeling left out can be dealt with only when we share them. If one or both of you have difficulty sharing painful feelings, now is the time to begin learning to open up. An easy way to start is to set aside several times a week when you can talk seriously together. Start getting in touch with your feelings by saying something like: "I feel (name the emotion) because (reasons)."

3. Know that there will be many well-intentioned people in your church, and even in your family, who will neither understand your feelings nor know how to help—unless they too have been through a struggle with infertility.

4. Take responsibility for your problem. Do not sit passively by and allow yourself to develop the attitude of "whatever will be will be." Treatment, both psychological and medical, is available.

*I didn't realize it then, but all those nights I
left Patricia sitting alone in the living room
while I went into my den to read were times
of running away.*

2
The Crises of
Infertility

INFERTILITY is a crisis of control. Whenever we feel that
we are no longer in control of what is happening to us,
we experience anxiety. As we struggle to conceive, we
find ourselves gradually losing control over many of the
most intimate aspects of our lives. We lose control of our
bodies as we discover that there are things going on inside
us over which we are powerless. We lose any sense of
control over the future, since we're no longer sure what the
future holds. Our marriage may become a roller-coaster ride
as the treatment process begins to build added tension
between ourselves and our partner.[1]

The Crisis of Emotions and Relationships

Patricia

Back then Alan hadn't learned to share his feelings very well. Whenever something bothered him he would just clam up, not saying anything. He would go into his den at night, shut the door, and read. I knew he was working on his seminar research, but I began to feel he was shutting me out. That was especially painful since I already felt left out by the women at church. They tried to include me and make me feel welcome, but I was, after all, different. They had children and I didn't.

I had become odd-woman-out to the world. Sometimes during the one-hour commute home from my office, my depression would get so bad I would cry all the way. Alan usually was out making calls or working on a paper when I got home, but whenever I was around him I tried to act like I was all right. Then I'd go stand in the shower and cry some more.

When I look back on that time, I remember a terribly overwhelming sense of having failed. Real women have babies. That's the message that seemed to come through every television commercial for diapers. The popular image of the '80s was the "supermom" who could do it all: have a sexually fulfilling, exciting marriage, an up-and-coming career, *and* be a mother. I tried to tell myself that two out of three wasn't bad, but the commercials and magazine ads about "mothers who do it all" let me know I was a failure.

Failure is almost always accompanied by guilt. The two are partners when it comes to emotions. *If I've failed at becoming a mother,* I reasoned, *it must be because I don't deserve to succeed.* So there had to be a reason I could not get pregnant—either I had done something terrible in my past, something I deserved to be punished for, or God knew that I didn't have what it takes to be a good mother.

Guilt. Failure. Feeling left out, defective. No wonder there were days when I cried at anything and everything that reminded me of what Alan and I did not have.

Alan

That's the way it is with infertility. Torrents of emotions may sweep over us at any time. The spouse who has the medical impairment is almost always flooded with feelings of failure and guilt. That person may question his or her maleness or femaleness. A woman may feel she's less than she should be since she is having difficulty giving her husband a child. If the medical problem is his, he may feel his manhood is in doubt because he cannot fulfill his role in the conception process.

Things are just as difficult for the spouse who doesn't have the physical problem. He or she is certain to experience not only depression, but also the anger and frustration of helplessness. One of the most painful aspects of a loving, caring relationship is watching your spouse suffer from something you can't do anything about. If the couple isn't careful, such frustration can lead to an emotional withdrawal, distancing one from the other just at the time support and understanding are needed most. This strain increases the stress already felt by the treatment process, and creates a vicious cycle that can lead to separation and divorce.

I didn't realize it then, but all those nights I left Patricia sitting alone in the living room while I went into my den to read were times of running away. Not that I didn't have work to do—I did. But many nights I would finish early, put on my headphones, and get lost in the music. The truth was, I didn't want to be reminded. What could I do, anyway? The more I noticed her depression, the more frustrated and angry I became.

There's little worse, I think, than being faced with a problem you can do nothing about. Having been in parish ministry for over a decade, I have learned that I really can't "fix" people when they are broken and hurting. The most I can do is enter their suffering with them, trying to bring God's presence however I can. I didn't understand that back then. My frustration stemmed from being unable to help Patricia. *I'm a minister! I'm supposed to know how to handle this!* I thought. And when I couldn't help, all I could feel was rage.

So I did what many spouses—especially men—do: I shut out the problem, buried myself in my work, and refused to even acknowledge what I was feeling. The distance between us grew. My wife's temperature chart dictated when we had sex. Neither of us talked very much about our feelings. There seemed to be an unspoken rule in the house forbidding our broaching the subject unless we absolutely had to. Emotional and physical exhaustion reduced our immunity and we both were sick a lot during that first year of treatment.

The Grief Process

What neither of us realized then was that couples in treatment go through a very real grief process. Guilt, frustration, anger, and depression are emotions that either overflow like a stream or get dammed up by a wall of denial. All these are part of the process of grieving. Unlike the loss of a person, though, infertility confronts us with the possible loss of a dream: the dream of having our own child, of a family life that may never be. And everyone knows you can never completely bury a dream.

Even so, setting our emotions and the stress they bring into our relationships within the context of the grief process—as we will do in the next chapter—may provide us with ways to understand and cope.

The Crisis of Faith

Patricia

Many times in our lives we turn to our faith as a source of comfort and hope. With the advent of a fertility crisis, however, the same faith we've turned to in the past often becomes a large part of the problem. We pray for the gift of a child, and it seems no one is listening. We may get the idea we are being punished for some past wrong. We look back over our lives and wonder what we could have done to cause God to visit such a plague upon us. Turning to the Scriptures we find stories of miraculous healing. *If God could heal then,* we think, *why isn't He willing to do the same for us now?*

Once I asked Alan if he thought the healings in the New Testament really took place. Maybe they were just stories after all. By now I was ending my second year of treatment, seeing an infertility specialist rather than my gynecologist, and taking clomid, a mild fertility drug prescribed to enhance ovulation. Like Sarah, Rachel, and Hannah—all my Old Testament counterparts—I had prayed more fervently than at any other time I can remember. But for what? It had now been two years of sex on schedule, expensive visits to the doctor's office and the drug store—and still nothing.

My childhood faith turned to bitter cynicism. Why pray when nothing happens? Hope was something other people had. I'd been hoping and praying for two years that my period wouldn't come and was disappointed every month. Why bother talking to a God who keeps letting you down?

Alan and I grew up in church. We were taught that God is just and loving. Yet where was the justice in this? Where was God's justice when thousands of teenagers got pregnant every year and we couldn't? We read the statistics on abortion, and were outraged to find there were so few infants available for adoption. You know the feeling. You turn on the evening news, see stories of child abuse, even murder, and wonder why God would even allow these people near children. It makes you want to throw something through the screen. So you ask yourself, *How can we believe in a God of love when we see so many abused, unwanted children in the world and we who would love a child so much ache with emptiness?* Our struggle of faith can be reduced to this one not-so-simple question: How can I understand God's love for my spouse and me in light of all this?

Alan

Later in the book we will wrestle with these challenges that infertility presents to our faith. And we will gain a deeper level of understanding both of ourselves and of God, God's love for us, and how God apparently does and does not choose to work in our lives.

The Crisis of Moral Choices

When we consider the host of options modern medical science now offers the infertile couple, we must realize that these alternatives are not without moral implications. They demand we answer questions that are new to us—questions about when life begins, and what is or isn't acceptable to us in our quest to bear a child.

In vitro fertilization, for example, asks us to make an informed decision about when life begins. This process involves taking eggs from the female and placing them in a glass dish with sperm, hoping that at least one egg will be fertilized. With this method it is not unusual for more than one egg to be impregnated. Three or four of the fertilized eggs are then injected into the uterus in the hope that one will attach itself to the uterine wall and begin to grow.

This presents us with a moral dilemma: What is to be done with those fertilized eggs that will not be used? If we believe life begins at conception, when sperm and egg unite, are we then committing murder by throwing away the unused eggs? Or does life begin at implantation, when the fertilized egg attaches itself to the uterine wall and begins to grow toward the embryo stage?

What of artificial insemination, using sperm from a donor rather than from the husband? How will you, the wife, feel about carrying a child not conceived from your husband's sperm? How will you, her husband, feel? Does this constitute some strange sort of adultery, even though no sexual exchange has taken place?

What of the much-publicized surrogate motherhood, where a woman carries a child whom she will at birth hand over to another couple? The legal and ethical questions surrounding this extraordinary practice, as ancient as the

Old Testament and as contemporary as today's headlines, are extremely complex. Chapter 10 may help you decide how you feel about the surrogacy option.

What about adoption? Is it right for us? How do we know we can love a child we didn't conceive? And what if we should adopt and then become pregnant? Will we feel differently about our "natural" child? Will this create hostility or alienation between them as they grow up? When should we start trying to adopt? And what if a child becomes available before we've exhausted all our options to conceive by natural means?

These and other questions call us to examine seriously what we believe about conception, parenting, and the place a child may or may not have in our lives. They prompt us to search ourselves deeply and prayerfully, for God's will— not just God's will in general, but God's will for us as potential parents.

However traumatic our pain, however great our desperation, we cannot afford to ignore the moral questions presented by our quest to have a child. We must be fearlessly and sometimes painfully honest with ourselves, our partner, and our God. Difficult though that may be, without such honesty we risk making decisions we cannot live with. We can do little to ourselves that is more destructive than to make a decision that contradicts our own values.

Conclusion

Infertility is a handicap, an impairment of the body's natural reproductive capacity. If you are to cope effectively with it, you must begin to realize what this means. Above all you must understand this is not something you brought willingly upon yourself. You did not choose to be infertile any more than you could choose to have appendicitis. You are not responsible for having a handicap.

You are responsible, however, for learning how to cope with it and overcome it. You are responsible for seeking the best medical help available and for struggling openly, even creatively, with your emotions, your relationship with your spouse, and your faith. You are responsible for the decisions you make about entering and continuing treatment and for getting counseling when the emotional burdens become more than you can bear. Your responsibility also includes the moral decisions you will make regarding alternatives to natural conception.

In addition, you are responsible for choosing your attitude toward the struggle. Attitude is crucial. You can say, "I will not allow my handicap to destroy me, nor will I allow it to destroy my marriage."

You cannot control what is happening in your body. You cannot determine the outcome of the treatment process. You may be able to influence in a helpful way, but you cannot control the way your spouse responds to you and to what happens between you. However, you *can* decide how *you* will handle whatever happens.

Every crisis, even the illness or death of your closest loved one, is a two-sided coin. One side is the pain of loss, because in every crisis something very precious to us is lost. In the case of infertility, it is the loss of a dream, of a hope, of a child that for you may never be. Yet this is only one side of the coin.

The other side is the opportunity for growth. The crisis of infertility can defeat you and ruin the rest of your life, or it can be something you "grow through" to a deeper understanding of yourself and your faith, and to a greater commitment to your partner. Growth or defeat is largely a matter of inner decision.

Decide today that, whatever happens, you can and will cope effectively with the outcome. Decide you will "grow through" this crisis, just the way you've managed to grow through others you've faced. Know that the coin of pain, inner conflict, and faith struggle does have another side. Resolution will come. It may or may not be what you hope for, but it will come. Either you will conceive and bear a child or you won't. You will adopt, or you will choose to remain childless and get on with your life. There is an end to the struggle. Sometimes this is all you have to hang on to. If this is where you are right now, then hang on to that.

THINGS TO DO

1. Decide to contend for your faith. At times all the great men and women of the Bible felt the lack of God's presence. They felt God had abandoned them but they still trusted He would see them through whatever crises they faced.

2. Decide that you will not withdraw from the world outside your door. Anxiety, depression, or marital stress can make you want to hide from life, but that only makes things worse. Keep up your activities. Be with people. Exercise—it releases the body's natural anti-depressants.

3. Be good to yourself. Treat yourself with respect. Don't allow yourself to slip into the trap of negative, self-deprecating thoughts. Affirm your basic goodness, your essential worth as a child of God. Remind yourself that when "God so loved the world that He gave

His only begotten Son," He had *you* in mind. Understand that God loves you, even if you don't feel His love at this time in your life.

4. If one is available, join a Resolve group in your area. Founded by Barbara Eck Menning, Resolve is a support group for infertile couples. Check with your infertility specialist's office—they usually know whether there is a local chapter of Resolve.

5. If communication and intimacy appear bogged down in your marriage, find a therapist or minister who understands the dynamics of the infertility struggle and go for counseling. Things can get much better when you learn to deal with the stress and to communicate more effectively with each other.

*Infertile couples often develop a vicious cycle
of emotional closeness and then withdrawal.
It is a roller-coaster existence.*

3
Why Do I Feel
This Way?

Alan

I HAD BEEN sitting in the surgery waiting room for about
two hours when our infertility specialist came in. "Everything went fine," he said. "She'll be ready to go home in
a couple of hours." He had just completed Patricia's first
laparoscopy, a minor surgical procedure that allows the
doctor to look inside the reproductive system to see
whether there might be any abnormalities or disease.

"There were some lesions that were probably due to her
ruptured appendix; also the fallopian tubes were kinked a
bit, but I think I straightened those out. So what we'll do is
increase the clomid dosage and wait a few more months."

Finally we were getting somewhere. Nothing serious
was wrong. Nothing minor surgery and a few more months
of pills wouldn't cure, anyway.

Patricia

When Alan explained what the doctor had found, I felt relieved, but cautious. It had been two years of ups and downs. After that you're very careful about getting your hopes up. You get tired of being let down. Still, I couldn't help but think this was it. A few more months and I'd be pregnant and taking childbirth classes.

But then weeks of waiting turn into months of disappointment. I tried my best to fight off the negative moods, but the depression gradually crept back into every crevice of my life. Then the doctor began talking about another, more extensive operation. This time I'd be in the hospital for a week. I wanted to hope but I was afraid to. I didn't want to go through that again. Yet I couldn't give up, not just now. Something inside kept telling me to take the next step up the treatment ladder—this time might be different. So I found myself living in a dull, gray world where hope and depression joined hands as my constant companions.

Infertility is an emotional roller coaster. Some days you're on top of the world. The doctor changes your medication, so you tell yourself this will surely be the wonder drug that does the trick. Or you leave the hospital after surgery. Once again life looks brighter because certainly the problem is corrected. Deep inside you feel you are only a few months away from holding your dream child in your arms.

Then it doesn't happen and eventually you begin to have doubts about your marriage. A coldness develops between you and your spouse. Conversation becomes minimal, polite but superficial; each of you seems to be trying to hide something. Tension builds. Instead of marriage partners, you begin to wonder if you aren't just two people sharing a house and paying rent out of the same checkbook.

Alan

Infertile couples often develop a vicious cycle of emotional closeness and withdrawal. With every new treatment there is renewed hope. Hope relieves some of the anxiety, making it easier to experience and share that emotional intimacy that makes a marriage work. But as hope fades, depression, anger, and frustration all creep back into the relationship and we withdraw from one another all over again.

The grief process of infertility has an unusual twist that makes it even more difficult to cope with than the death of a family member or a friend. When someone close to you dies there is a tangible loss. Your friend is no longer present—the funeral marks the passage from living with this person to living without him. And we are expected to mourn. It's healthy. Friends and family give their support because they understand and appreciate what we're going through.

This isn't the case for the infertile couple. Unless your case is hopeless from the start, you may live with a strange mixture of grief *and* hope. You mourn because you have no child, yet you hang on to the hope of conception. It's this joining of grief and hope that makes infertility so painful. We grieve over the loss of *potential* rather than the loss of something actual. We mourn the loss of a biological heir, of the pregnancy and birth experience, the wonders of breast feeding, and the joys of parenting. These are all very real losses to the infertile couple.

In our first parsonage there was a small bedroom off one side of the hallway. It was clearly meant to be a nursery, but for Patricia and me it was just an empty room that served as a daily reminder.

Patricia

One afternoon one of the men from the church was helping Alan move some old furniture into that room. I was supervising. When they finished, this friend, with no intention of being cruel, looked at me and said, "You know, this little room will make you a nice nursery someday."

I was stunned. The emptiness in the pit of my stomach was almost unbearable.

No one seemed to understand. Our friends did not comfort us because they didn't see infertility as any kind of loss. Rather, most of them told us to "just keep trying." That was the last thing I needed to hear, and it made Alan furious, even though we both understood they meant no harm. So we were left to work through our grief alone.

Alan

It's important to remember that grief *is* something we all have to *work* through. It doesn't just magically go away after a few weeks or months. There is actually a grief process that we can divide into stages to help us better cope with our feelings, and for infertile couples they are experienced in a unique way.

Infertility and the Grief Process

According to Elizabeth Kubler-Ross, healthy mourning requires us to move through the stages of grief. At first there is denial, followed by anger, bargaining, depression, and finally, acceptance.

Before we examine the grief process in detail, we want you to stop for a moment to reflect on how you may have dealt with other crises in your life. Each of us has a repertoire of coping skills we've developed over the years. Now is the time to look within and pull out those that have served you well in the past.

Begin by asking yourself some questions. What activities enabled you to relieve your anxiety? Was there a trusted friend, who wasn't involved in the crisis itself, with whom you could share your deepest feelings, your fears? Did you go for counseling?

Nothing is more important in the healing process than finding someone with whom you can be honest about your feelings.

While I was at school I stayed in the home of the professor who was chairman of my doctoral committee. We had come to Louisville the same year—he as a professor, I as a first-year M.Div. student. We car-pooled for years and became good friends. Bill was my mentor, pastor, teacher, and fellow struggler in the faith. More than once we sat up late at night as he listened to me vent my frustration. He was among the first of my friends and colleagues who have helped me in the long process of getting in touch with my true feelings. It's like venting a volcano. You have to find a constructive way to let off the pressure occasionally or you'll explode.

You need a friend, someone outside your marriage, to talk with. But we want to offer a word of caution. Since infertility is not something everyone experiences, friends and family might not be able to identify with what you're going through. Pick your confidants cautiously. You need someone who will hear you, someone who will help you get in touch with and express your feelings in a non-threatening environment. Avoid like the plague anyone who offers unsolicited advice or who tends to attach moral judgments to feelings. Such people, well-meaning though they may be, can cause you more emotional trauma than you can imagine.

Emotions are powerful, threatening at times to overwhelm us. We fear that if we honestly express them they may destroy us. The truth is just the opposite. It is when we don't allow our feelings to come out into the open where we can deal with them that they become harmful. So as you read through these stages, keep one eye on the page and another on your emotions. When something sounds familiar, let yourself identify the feeling, and experience it to the fullest. Our hurts can be healed. But first we have to acknowledge the pain.

Stage One: Denial

Patricia

After trying to get pregnant for about a year I began to suspect something was wrong. Alan didn't see it that way. He was almost sure there couldn't be. I was healthy in every other way. So he kept pushing the subject aside every time I'd bring it up. At the time I thought he was just trying to be encouraging. Now I recognize that it was his way of refusing to deal with even the possibility that I might have a real medical problem.

Denial can persist for months or years because there is so much at stake. Infertility threatens many of the most intimate facets of our lives. Self-esteem takes a beating. Being a "real man" or "real woman" means, so we're taught to think, being able to procreate. Our natural inclination is to discount all the evidence because we do not want to experience the trauma of not being a real man or woman.

For some, denial manifests itself in frantic running from doctor to doctor, hoping for a different diagnosis. While it's good to get a second or maybe even a third opinion, we eventually need to stop running and face facts. When specialist after specialist tells us the same story, it's a good bet that denial has gone on long enough.

Others, particularly men, lose themselves in their work, hiding behind busy schedules and a multitude of tasks, but eventually they must confront the harsh reality of the situation.

Slowly the wall of denial begins tumbling down and the truth seeps over the top. You or your spouse, or maybe even both of you, have a fertility problem. You have wanted children, planned for them, even prayed for them. Now you begin to accept the possibility that you may never conceive one of your own. Allowing these thoughts into your awareness and experiencing the pain they bring with them is one sign that denial may be subsiding.

Stage Two: Anger

Driving down the street I noticed a mother severely scolding her toddler for leaving her doll carriage in the driveway. Suddenly, from out of nowhere, there came a fury the likes of which I'd rarely experienced. I felt like ripping the steering wheel off the column. I wanted to slam on the brakes, get out and yell, "For God's sake! Don't you know how lucky you are? How dare you treat this child like that?"

That's anger. And if this, or something like it, has happened to you, then you are already acquainted with the second stage of grief. Anger is a very natural response to loss of control. We get angry with ourselves, our doctors, our spouse, our relatives, God, the dog, the cat, and just about everything else.

Why? Because infertility gives us plenty to be angry about. We're angry because we feel loss, because we're hurt and afraid, because we feel trapped by circumstances beyond our control. The tension builds inside until we reach the boiling point, exploding at any convenient target. Knowing the losses are only potential losses doesn't help much. Deep inside we fear our worst nightmares will come true. The smallest marital problems may awaken fears that our spouse will leave us because the infertility somehow makes us defective. Or, if it's our spouse who has the problem, we may feel cheated, even wronged, knowing we could have had a child if we had just married someone else.

Suffering all these hurts and fears, who wouldn't be angry?

Recognize these many faces of anger. Learn to identify them in yourself and in your marriage and in your relationships with family and co-workers. Anger recognized can be managed. Unrecognized, it can wreck your marriage, spoil other significant relationships, and drive you into serious depression.

Many of us grew up being told it was wrong to express anger. So we forced it underground, learned to control it, kept it under wraps. Some of us learned our lessons so well that we're no longer even aware we're angry. Instead of rage, what we now feel is depression, or a dull numbness that is almost devoid of any feeling. Of course, the thing about anger—and many other emotions—is that no matter how hard you try, you can't make it stay underground.

Sooner or later anger will surface, and it will find a target. If you are the type of person who hasn't learned how to deal appropriately with anger, you may become the proverbial "loose cannon," firing at whatever moves. Doctors are a favorite target, especially in the early months of treatment. We expect them to be miracle workers. Discovering there are no quick fixes, we may lash out at the physician who is doing his best to help.

As a general rule, when you find yourself overreacting to something that really isn't that big a deal, like your spouse being late for dinner or burning the toast, it's a good bet you're really angry about something else.

With infertility, the real target of your anger is the situation. Problem is, situations aren't something we can attack directly. There is nothing "out there," no person, no object to hit or get mad at. So we do the next best thing: we vent our rage at people, or the dog, or the vacuum cleaner that isn't working properly. Soon we get around to being angry with God. Since the doctor can't be held responsible, and being angry with our spouse threatens our marriage, then God must be the one to blame. So we aim all of our frustration at the Creator. After all, God controls everything, right?

Before we go further, let us say we believe it's not only okay to be angry with God, but it's also psychologically and spiritually healthy. So if you really want healing for your battered emotions, you need to grant yourself the privilege of being angry with God.

Be assured God is big enough to accept your anger without being hostile in return. The biblical witness tells us "nothing can separate us from His love." Anger at God is nothing to feel guilty about. And prayer is a great place to vent your hostilities. Allow your outrage to boil up and explode in God's direction. After a while you'll feel better for it. It's a great tension release that may keep you from victimizing innocent people. And, if you're patient, your angry prayers may lead you into a faith deeper than any you've known before.

What is most dangerous is directing anger inward, against yourself. The mistaken notion that infertility is somehow your fault—which it isn't—can cause you to lay loads of self-blame on your already burdened spirit. It's easy to get down on yourself.

No matter how many times Alan would tell me that I'd done nothing to deserve any of this, I would always come back with, "Of course it's my fault. It must be. There's no one else left to blame. I must have done something to cause this! If I weren't such a terrible person, none of this would be happening. I guess God knows I'd make a terrible mother!"

Self-blame is dangerous to our emotional and physical health. Anger turned inward, unresolved, misdirected, leads down a slippery slope into a sea of depression. If you aren't careful you may drown there. When you discover you are living daily with self-blame, or find you are carrying a huge burden of guilt because you think God is punishing you for something, then it's time to seek professional help.

Unless you genuinely accept that infertility is a disease for which you are not responsible, your self-blame will push you ever more deeply into the depression. That can adversely impact your physical, emotional, and spiritual health and your marriage, and may even reduce your chances of conception.

Stage Three: Bargaining

When Alan and I were in college and seminary, I had every intention of having both a career and a family. And of course there's nothing wrong with doing both. These days many women, even young mothers, work outside the home. It's almost an economic necessity. But as my treatment wore on I found myself promising God that I would not only quit work but give up entirely on having a career if only He would answer our prayers for a baby.

When the energy of rage begins to dissipate we usually enter the bargaining stage. If God hasn't responded to our angry pleas, we think, then maybe He will be more favorable if we play "let's make a deal." We will pledge almost anything. People promise to go into the ministry or dedicate themselves more fully to Christian service—if only God will grant their wish for a child.

We learn our bargaining skills at an early age. When a young child discovers temper tantrums are ineffective she will change her tactics, promising to put all of her toys back into the playpen if only Mom will let her play outside.

This behavior carries over into adulthood. It's a way of trying to get what you want from another person, or even from God.

Bargaining is frequently related to guilt. When things aren't going well we feel we are somehow at fault. Everyone can look back and see things done or left undone that we aren't very proud of. We are imperfect creatures, and during this stage all our flaws stand out like sore thumbs. So it isn't surprising that we would make promises to clean up our lives, or never to do this or that again, if only God would grant our wish.

We will talk more about this in Chapter 7, but let me say for now that God is not like Santa Claus. He does not keep a list of who's been naughty and who's been nice so He can hand out presents to good little boys and girls. God withholds neither grace nor children from those who have sinned and fallen short of what He created us to be. Just looking around at some of the people who have children should be enough to convince anyone of this truth. Many parents have histories much darker than ours, and some are just plain bad parents. Many even abuse their children. We need to realize that neither moral purity nor consistent church attendance are prerequisites demanded by God in return for pregnancy.

Stage Four: Depression

Depression sets in after bargaining has failed, stealing whatever joy you have been able to hang on to as you struggled through treatment after treatment, month after month. Depression is a natural result of loss. And with infertility there is much to lose.

Whenever someone close to you dies, there is that experience of intense mourning between the time we're notified of the death and the funeral. I remember feeling that way for months on end, like something inside me had died. And in a way it had. I had lost the pregnancy and birth experience, my self-image as a woman and a wife.

Before our infertility crisis, Alan and I had dreams of playing ball in the backyard with our toddler and of trips to the zoo on Saturday afternoons. All those things now seemed meant for someone else. It seemed as though our future had died. After all, if we weren't going to be dual-career parents, then what would we be? Up to that point, part of our self-image had been formed by a mental concept of fatherhood and motherhood. Taking away those roles left us with visions of growing old alone, the last of our respective families.

When our self-image is so radically altered, it's no wonder we feel depressed. We have lost a vital facet of our personal identity. It may sound trite, but it's true. In the midst of an infertility crisis, we no longer know with any certainty just who we are or where we're going with our lives.

This stage is all the more difficult because much of what we see every day can trigger anything from a mild case of the blues to a bout with depression serious enough to leave you bedridden. You notice a young mother pushing a stroller through the grocery store, and a pervasive sense of gloom seems to wrap around you like a fog. Mother's Day. Father's Day. Thanksgiving. Christmas. Any holiday may leave you feeling down for weeks before and weeks afterward.

Though painful, depression is a necessary step on the path to acceptance. And no matter how much we try, there is really no healthy way to short-circuit the grief process without risking severe damage to our emotional well-being and physical health. The sense of quiet despair, the physical and mental lethargy accompanied by the many bodily symptoms of distress, all are unpleasant facets of mourning that we need to experience so we can cleanse the sorrow from our lives and get on with the business of living.

Normal depression doesn't last very long—a few weeks at most. But what if your depression has hung on for months? If you or your partner fall into that category, then what you are experiencing may not be normal depression. Barbara Eck Menning writes:

> Pathological depression is a smoke screen behind which much more powerful and frightening feelings lurk. Inability to address anger, guilt, or grief can lead to repression of these natural and necessary feelings. A chronic depression can ensue that may continue indefinitely until the real feelings are acknowledged.[1]

This is the high price we may end up paying should we get into the habit of suppressing our true feelings.

Uncovering feelings buried long ago is always scary. There are times when we need the help of a trained professional to peel back the layers of our soul, to free us from our fear of hurting too much. A therapist can enable you to sort out the various emotions your depression may be masking, as well as help you summon the courage to face them. Don't be afraid to ask for professional assistance when you need it. Facing deeply rooted anxieties will be painful. But it's far more destructive to leave them just below the surface, unacknowledged and therefore unresolved. In a way, therapy is like a trip to the dentist's office. You know it will hurt for a little while, but the pain is necessary to keep the abscess from poisoning your whole system.

Stage Five: Acceptance

Acceptance is the last stage of the grief process. In acceptance you are neither angry nor depressed. You have vented your hostilities and worked through many of your feelings. It's more a state of emotional, mental, and physical exhaustion than anything else. Feelings fall somewhere between happy and sad, usually a blend of both.

After almost five years of operations, tests, and treatments, now we knew the score. We knew there was still an outside chance for conception but we had finally reached the stage where our specialist told us there was nothing else he could do. We were forced to admit we probably would never have the child we had longed for, prayed for all these years. We had come to the place where we had to make a conscious decision to cope with our predicament as best we could and get on with living.

It wasn't that we were giving up, not entirely anyway. The doctor had said there was still a chance, however slim. If we wanted to consider adoption, then this was the time to start applying to the agencies. If not, then we needed to work on redefining our roles and building a life together as a childless couple. There was a real sense of sadness, but also of relief. No more operations, injections of pergonal, temperature charts, or sex on schedule. Slowly we were able to accept what had happened, realize how devastating our experience had been to each of us and to our relationship, and get on with our lives.

Acceptance may be a resolution, in which case you and your partner begin working on a life without children or decide to start adoption proceedings. Or it may be a time to evaluate your options and decide whether to continue treatment, which means running the risk of experiencing another cycle of the grief process. Or you may decide to investigate one of the many alternatives to traditional conception currently offered by medical science.

At this point infertility differs from most other grief experiences. As we said earlier, the loss of a friend through death has a certain finality to it that is absent in infertility.

There are no funerals to mark the loss of a *potential* child, no ritual to help heal the hurt that comes from knowing you may never feel the pain and joy of the delivery room. Infertile couples must learn to live with their grief, knowing that occasionally some of the feelings common to the grief process will return.

One Mother's Day about a year after I had discontinued treatment was particularly difficult. The church had a tradition of giving flowers to all the mothers during the worship service. It was all I could do to keep from running out when someone—without intending to be cruel—gave me a flower. I was the only non-mother walking around with a little potted plant. The feeling of being different, like everyone knew there was something wrong with me but nobody wanted to mention it, all came back. Once more I needed to work through the feelings.

When things like that happen, you may feel like the psalmist who asked, "How long, O Lord, how long?" Like the psalmist, you will need to reach through your pain to grasp the hand of God, praying for understanding, strength, and hope. You will need to make a conscious, willful decision to again turn your life over to God's care, trusting that, just like the last time, He will see you through.

Grief *will* return from time to time. There is really nothing you can do to prevent it. Understand that this is natural, that you can and will work through the feelings, and that you can reach an even deeper level of acceptance and faith.

THINGS TO DO

1. Try to pinpoint where you are in the grief process. This is the first step in working through the various emotions associated with that phase.

2. Fully admit your feelings into your consciousness. Repressed emotions will do more damage to you and to your relationships than you can imagine.

3. Read as much as you can on the grief process and how to deal with it. The more you understand about what you are feeling and why, the better you will be able to cope with it.

4. Stay "emotionally in touch" with your spouse. Too often we tend to "walk on eggs" in our marriage for fear of hurting the other person or starting an argument. That leads to emotional distancing, loss of intimacy, and potentially serious marital problems. Let each other know exactly how you are feeling.

Just when we need each other most,
the distance between us grows.

4

For Better or Worse

WE ENTER marriage with certain expectations, the most fundamental being that at some time in the course of our relationship we will have one or more children. Few couples marry with the intention of remaining childless, and of those who do, many change their minds as the years go by.

Alan

Like almost everyone else, Patricia and I assumed we would have a child when the time was right—after we had both finished school and gotten our respective careers under way. Putting off having children until their late twenties or early thirties is a common pattern for couples today. But by then most of us feel a certain pressure to enter this next stage of our lives.

Psychologist Erik Erikson's pioneering work indicates that we move through various "life stages" on our journey from cradle to grave, and he illustrates the importance of our desire to reproduce. Each stage has its own agenda.

The young adult stage, when we are most likely to begin thinking about a family, Erikson calls "generativity." The primary task here is to contribute something of yourself to life. It is a desire to create, to leave a legacy for the future. The way many of us choose to fulfill this task—though it certainly isn't the only way—is through having children.

When this basic need is stifled through infertility, we experience what Erikson calls "stagnation," primarily a sense of being cut off from the future. Thus we can understand why infertility brings a sense of sadness deep inside. We know that without offspring the family line, or at least our branch of it, will end with us.

This is hardly a novel idea. The ancient Hebrews of the Old Testament believed the life of the father and mother were continued through their children. Not having children, particularly male children, meant one's influence would end at death, something every Hebrew feared.

Both the ancient Judeo-Christian tradition and contemporary psychology underscore the importance of procreation. Each gives us insight into why even those who enter marriage without intending to have children later change their minds as they sense their biological clocks winding down.

We would hasten to add, however, that this does not mean *every* couple must have children any more than it means every individual should get married. Still less should this be interpreted as saying those who do not marry and reproduce have no chance for growing toward mature, fulfilling adulthood. Such sweeping generalizations are bound to be false. Jesus, for example, neither married nor had children. If we take the New Testament seriously, then we must believe Jesus was as fulfilled, as mature, as complete as any human being could possibly be.

The Hebraic emphasis on parents living through their children and psychology's concept of generativity each points to one of our primary needs as men and women created in the image of God: the need to contribute something of ourselves to the great unfolding drama of human history. None of us wants to vanish without a trace. We want to leave a marker, something with our name on it that lets those who follow know we have passed this way, that life is better for our having been here. Children, for many of us, become the most significant means through which we try to fulfill this basic desire.

Those who are single, either by choice or through lack of a suitable partner, and those whose desire for children has been stymied by infertility must find other ways to pursue this innate creative impulse. Infertility, traumatic and devastating as it may be, does not decree the end of a meaningful existence.

In addition to these internal creative pressures, family and society place the burden of their expectations on us. Our parents expect us to give them grandchildren. Our siblings expect that we will honor them with a niece or nephew. Friends expect us to accompany them on the journey through parenthood.

With all these pressures, within and without, it's easy to understand how the desire to parent can quickly turn into an obsession. Infertility sets a roadblock between ourselves and one of life's important goals. Is it any wonder all this has a tremendous impact on our marriage?

This is particularly true when you are the one with the medical problem. My wife felt she had failed me—no matter how much I told her otherwise—because she could not give her husband a child. Feelings of low self-worth usually cause you to draw back into yourself. Communication breaks down and putting on a front, smiling when you feel like crying, eventually becomes exhausting.

When Patricia was going through all this I became frustrated and angry. None of us likes to see the one we love most suffer. I wanted to offer support. I wanted to assure her that she hadn't failed me, that I loved her no less than before. Yet I found it increasingly difficult to penetrate her wall of depression. Wanting to help and not knowing how, or being unable to help even when I did, left me feeling more and more isolated from her pain.

Looking back, I realize we had developed the pattern common to infertile couples where the spouse with the medical problem gets depressed and feels worthless and the partner wants to help but ends up feeling frustrated. Just when we need each other most, the distance between us grows. Little annoyances turn into big problems and the specter of infertility becomes the unseen guest at every meal, an unwanted intruder in the bedroom.

If you are the husband and the medical problem is yours, you may be experiencing these same feelings of failure and worthlessness: that your masculinity is threatened, that you aren't a "real man," or that you are a failure sexually. These feelings can be all the more intense because, like most men, you are hesitant about reaching out for emotional support when you need it. Anger builds up inside: anger at yourself, anger at those who don't want to understand, anger that can spill over into your marriage if you aren't careful.

Performance Anxiety

Doubts about sexual prowess, complicated by the need to have intercourse on schedule, lead many men to experience performance anxiety. Some men experience a loss of sexual desire, or even temporary impotence.[1]

We men react to all this much the same as our spouses, becoming depressed and withdrawn. The more support she tries to offer, the more we are unable to respond. This may lead to another common pattern that develops with infertile couples: "the hysterical wife and the silent husband."

It works like this. She loves you. She wants to be supportive, to assure you of her love, to tell you she's not planning to leave just because you have this problem. So she reaches out to you in every way she knows how.

But with your macho image threatened, you already feel inadequate as husband and lover, so you don't want to talk about any of it. It's embarrassing. It makes you angry, threatened because you can't control any of what's happening to you. So the more she reaches out, the more you withdraw into your own little shell. After a while she can't help but get frustrated by your unwillingness to communicate, so she stops trying and the distance between you grows.

As you might well imagine, all this has a profound effect on a couple's sex life.

Infertility treatments do demand a certain amount of "sex on schedule." And this can make sex very depersonalized, robbing intercourse of spontaneity and emotional support. The danger comes from letting your sex life be reduced to *nothing more* than sex on schedule.

Just because you are going through infertility treatments doesn't mean your sex life has to suffer. The idea is to try to keep it as normal as possible. Remember that making love is not just a physical act designed to result in children. Lovemaking is much more than the reproductive act. Nurture your relationship by taking time to enjoy each other sexually, with as little thought as possible about making babies. Tell each other what you need, emotionally and physically. Try some new positions. Take showers together. Do whatever you need to do to keep your sex life spontaneous and joyful. This will make those times when you "have to do it" a lot more fun.

When one or both of you are suffering loss of self-esteem, make the effort "to build one another up in love," as the apostle Paul says. Show your partner he or she is valued as a person, not merely as a necessary adjunct to procreation.

Above all, do not let communication break down completely. Be honest first with yourself, then don't be afraid to be honest with your partner. Learn as much as you can about what you are going through and why. Understanding and honesty are the two most important tools for coping with infertility.

Know that this crisis will have an end—whether you conceive, adopt, or remain childless. Whatever happens, you and your mate will one day regain the sense of control over your lives and your marriage that you lost when all this began. Knowing that resolution will come and that your relationship will not suffer interminably under this strain will help keep you going. You'll be able to manage when the bridge between you seems to have collapsed under the emotional burden of sex on schedule, temperature charts, and trips to the doctor's office.

As we come to the close of this chapter, we can imagine what you and your spouse are feeling—probably, overwhelmed. You knew something was wrong, that you felt disillusioned and down on yourself. You had no idea infertility could cause all this personal pain and marital discord. You may even feel you can't make it, but you can and will if you are willing to do what it takes. You and your spouse can come through this together.

By yourself you don't have the resources to cope with it all. The good news is, you don't have to make it alone. Support groups can help. Counseling can help. The two of you can learn to struggle across the emotional distances and help each other. And there is always the resource of personal faith.

If you are at all religious, you have probably tried faith already. And if you are like many infertile couples, you may think it hasn't helped much. Your faith may have become more of a problem, even a burden, than anything else. I know how that feels. More than once I exploded in rage at the God who allowed this kind of thing to happen. I quit believing entirely and then got angry because I couldn't stop believing. I abandoned belief in a just God the week I had to counsel a teenager who'd had an abortion while my wife was having another operation. The truth is, infertility can become as devastating to faith as it is to our personal and marital health.

Yet faith can become a resource. The Scriptures can help. Infertility can become a crisis that brings you to a deeper understanding of yourself, of God and His love, and of the true meaning of your marriage.

THINGS TO DO

1. Now is the time to take honest stock of your marriage. Sit down and make a list of the ways you think the infertility has affected it. Talk openly and honestly about each item on the list.

2. Do you feel closer or further apart as a couple than you did six months ago?

3. Do either or both of you withdraw into your own little world to keep from hurting or making the other angry?

4. Do you fall into the pattern of the silent partner and the hysterical spouse?

5. If, after discussing these questions, you see that you are drifting apart under the strain of it all, then by all means get help. Find a trained, certified therapist or minister skilled in marriage counseling—preferably one who understands the dynamics of infertility crises—and go.

6. Know that for counseling to help *both* of you it will take a commitment from *both* of you.

7. If your spouse will not go, then go by yourself. He or she may be persuaded to join you later. And even if that doesn't happen, you will learn more effective ways to help you deal with the situation.

When God's will for us is thwarted by the disease of infertility, Scripture gives us God's ultimate hope for our lives.

5
What Scripture Has to Tell Us

Patricia

I F YOU grew up in church as we did, chances are you came to believe certain things. Sunday school taught you about the God of infinite love who wanted only the best for His children, and about Jesus who went around healing the sick. You learned the Bible could be relied on as a guide leading to deeper faith and a better understanding of life.

Moving into adulthood you came to expect certain things from your faith. You learned to pray, trusting that God in His goodness and mercy would answer your prayers. During difficult times you depended on your faith to give you strength and courage to face those hard challenges. Like most people, you grew to believe that life was governed by divine justice, the idea that if you were moral, continued to grow in faith, and participated in the fellowship of Christ's church, then God's blessings would flow to you.

Now, in the midst of what may be the greatest crisis you have yet encountered, you may find many of these cherished beliefs overshadowed by doubt. Infertility, like an emotional earthquake, has shaken and begun to crack the foundations of your spiritual life.

For example, you may wonder why, if Jesus actually did heal sick people, your prayers for conception remain unanswered. Having searched the Scriptures from Genesis to Revelation, you may be baffled to discover that, with the exception of Michal in 2 Samuel 6:23, there are no permanently infertile couples mentioned in all those pages. If that weren't already discouraging enough, you may have run across passages like 1 Samuel 1:5, where Hannah, wife of Elkanah, is referred to as one who "the Lord kept from having children." So you wonder, *Is God keeping us from having a baby? If so, why? Have we done something terribly wrong? Are my spouse and I being punished?*

Faith itself becomes a problem for infertile couples. One Sunday at church a man came up to me and said, "You know, if God wants the two of you to have a child, you'll get one. You just need to keep trusting and praying."

I felt crushed. We had been doing just that for years. What hurt even more was the presupposition that seemed to lie behind that well-intentioned but painful remark: the idea that God sits up on high somewhere and doles out favors according to some merit system. The good boys and girls get what they want while the bad ones don't get anything. When you get this kind of jab at your self-esteem, you can't help but question your beliefs about God's goodness, the way God works in our lives, and the efficacy of prayer.

As we look now at some Bible stories of couples who experienced infertility, we will discover why women like Sarah, Hannah, and Rachel interpreted their barrenness as God's direct will. We also will see why you and I, by faith, can view infertility through more enlightened eyes. Scripture gives us God's ultimate hope for our lives, and shows us how we can turn to the Bible for comfort, strength, and renewal when God's will for us is thwarted by the disease of infertility.

Infertility and Scripture: A Look at Three Couples

In the first chapter of Genesis beginning with the 27th verse we read:

> So God created human beings, making them to be like himself. He created them male and female, blessed them, and said, "Have many children, so that your descendants will live all over the earth and bring it under their control."

While we shouldn't interpret this to mean every married couple *must* have children, we can reasonably conclude that these verses express God's intention for those who wish their union blessed with offspring. For most couples that's the way it works.

But if the Bible is anything, it is a very honest book about real people facing difficult situations, struggling with painful emotions, and wrestling with God to make some sense of their predicaments. In the Bible we find the stories of three infertile couples: Abraham and Sarah (Genesis

16:1–5), Jacob and Rachel (Genesis 30:1–2), and Elkanah and Hannah (1 Samuel 1:1–5).

Two significant details of these stories are worth noting. First, the problem appears always to be the woman's. She is the one regarded as "barren." There is never any question that it might be her husband's difficulty. The reason is rather easy to understand.

These passages date from a relatively primitive time. There was no science as we know it, no understanding comparable to ours of the way the human body works. As long as the man could ejaculate into the woman's vagina, he had done his part in the process. Hence if conception did not take place it must be because his wife was barren. She was forced to bear the full burden of their childlessness.

Second, and particularly disturbing to infertile couples, certain verses in each story seem to imply that God is directly, willfully responsible for the infertility. Sarah says to Abraham, "The Lord has kept me from having children" (Genesis 16:2). Jacob, angry with Rachel for her barrenness, says, "I can't take the place of God. He is the one who keeps you from having children" (Genesis 30:2). The author of 1 Samuel writes of Hannah, "the Lord kept her from having children" (1:5).

Are we, then, to believe *our* infertility is the result of God's will? Is divine intervention behind our predicament, our pain? Despite these verses, we believe you would be doing yourselves and your Creator a great disservice by shouldering God with this responsibility.

Abraham and Sarah, Jacob and Rachel, Elkanah and Hannah all viewed life through eyes unenlightened by modern medicine. They didn't understand about low sperm counts. They knew nothing of blocked fallopian tubes or hormonal imbalances. They viewed their lives and their world very differently from the way you and I do.

Most important for our discussion is their primitive understanding of God and His relationship to the world. Lacking any concept of physical handicaps or illnesses, these people believed God was responsible for whatever happened, be it good or bad. They believed in a righteous God who could be either pleased or angered by the moral choices of God's creatures. So if pregnancy occurred, it was regarded as a sign of God's blessing. When repeated attempts at conception failed, they felt—like many of today's infertile couples—cursed. Put all this together and it's not hard to see how a woman living in that day could be forced to endure her husband's blame and her own burden of shame as years went by and her infertility became apparent to everyone.

Unfortunately, vestiges of this thinking remain with us. More than once I have stood beside a hospital bed, listening to a patient wonder what he did wrong to deserve the pain of his illness. Occasionally I've run across those who believe the accidental death of a friend or relative was God's judgment on the victim's lifestyle.

So it's not uncommon for some of us to experience this kind of "punishment thinking" when deeply enmeshed in a fertility crisis. A man may wonder whether he's being punished because of an extramarital affair. A woman may feel guilty about her premarital sexual experience and wonder if God isn't making her pay the price for her sin.

Most of us already live with enough guilt. Some of it is legitimate, some probably isn't. What you and I do not need is an undeserved guilt trip. It is legitimate to feel a sense of guilt and shame if you have had an extramarital affair or engaged in a promiscuous lifestyle. It is not legitimate to let guilt push you into believing that God is punishing you by refusing to allow you and your spouse to conceive. We don't believe that God bears grudges; that's what forgiveness is all about. We need to realize that the Bible is a book whose main characters grow in understanding. Through their struggles, their triumphs and defeats, they are like infants whose eyesight gradually clears enough to see things as they really are. One generation builds on the understanding of another until God is no longer viewed as the divine rule-giver who repays everyone according to their rights and wrongs, but as the Divine Lover whose merciful kindness overflows even to those who sin against Him. Hence the writer of Psalm 103:10 could say:

> He does not punish us as we deserve or repay us according to our sins and wrongs.

And Jesus, when confronted with the woman who had been caught in the very act of adultery, told her: "I do not condemn you either. Go, but do not sin again" (John 8:11).

Of course, there is a sense in which infertility may be linked with certain sinful actions. If, for example, promiscuity leads to contracting a sexually transmitted disease that results in diminished fertility, then we can legitimately conclude that one's sin has resulted in infertility. *This is quite different from saying infertility is God's punishment for premarital sex or an extramarital affair.* It's one thing to say God has created a world in which we must bear the consequences of our actions, and quite another to say God causes something terrible to happen whenever we do something wrong.

Is God responsible for our infertility? Is childlessness the direct result of His will? No, we don't believe that, any more than we believe God's will is responsible for plane crashes or children being run over by drunk drivers.

We will deal more deeply with this in the next chapter, but for now let us agree that infertility is a physical handicap, a malfunction of the body's procreative system. Something has gone wrong with God's good creation so that the body no longer functions as God intended. The truth is, we live in a world where God's good intentions for us may sometimes be hindered. God is like any earthly father who wants only what is best for his children, but as any earthly father knows, things don't always work out the way we want them to.

Maturity: The Goal of Our Spiritual Journey

It will further help our understanding if we set the infertility experience within the larger context of God's ultimate hope for our lives. Paul writes to the Ephesians:

> And so we shall all come together to that oneness in faith and in our knowledge of the Son of God; we shall become *mature* people, reaching to the very height of Christ's full stature. Then we shall no longer be children, carried by the waves and blown about by every shifting wind of the teaching of deceitful men, who lead others into error by the tricks they invent. Instead, by speaking the truth in love, we must grow up in every way to Christ, who is the head. Under his control all the different parts of the body fit together by every joint with which it is provided. So when each separate part works as it should, the whole body grows and builds itself up through love (Ephesians 4:13–16).

Embroiled in the treatment process, struggling with grief, desperately clinging to any shred of hope, it becomes very difficult for us to maintain a Christian outlook on our

struggle. Conception often becomes an all-consuming pas-
sion. Many of us reach a point where we honestly believe
that without a child our lives will cease to have any meaning.

In the previous passage from Ephesians the apostle Paul
helps us regain a sense of Christian perspective. Children,
as much as we may desire them, as much as God might like
for us to have them, are not the be-all and end-all of our
Christian pilgrimage. The meaning of our lives does not
depend on our capacity to procreate any more than the
meaning of marriage lies in giving our parents grandchildren. Important as those things may be, they are not the
sole reasons for our existence.

So what is? Just what is the goal, the end of our striving
as men and women committed to the spiritual journey of
following Jesus Christ?

Paul writes that the goal of our lives, the meaning of our
existence, is that you and I should reach "that oneness in
faith and in our knowledge of the Son of God; *we shall
become mature people,* reaching to the very height of
Christ's full stature."

That word *mature* provides the key to understanding
God's ultimate hope for each of us. It comes from the Greek
word *teleo,* which means "to bring something to an end, to
complete something, to finish what was started." A mature
person, then, in the sense that Paul uses the term, would be
one who has become in every way Christlike, one who has
attained "the very height of Christ's full stature."

Obviously none of us has yet reached such lofty heights
of spiritual attainment. It's best to think of ourselves as men
and women "on the way" to maturity. So Paul encourages

us to "speak the truth in love," and to "grow up in every way to Christ, who is the head."

Mature personhood—becoming like Jesus Christ in every way—is the goal, the destination of our spiritual journey. It is what you and I are all about as men and women created in God's own image. And the way we grow toward that goal is by keeping Jesus Christ at the center of our lives, by focusing on Him and what He would have us do as His servants.

When struggling with infertility it's difficult to keep Christ at that vital center of our lives. The quest for conception can easily become an idolatrous concern, pushing Jesus Christ aside. This happens most often when we lose our Christian perspective as we are confronted with painful circumstances. Instead of praying for guidance to carry out God's will for our lives, our prayers may become little more than lengthy dissertations on our need to parent.

Or like Hannah, we may bargain with God, making promises that really aren't ours to make:

> Lord Almighty, look at me, your servant! See my trouble and remember me! Don't forget me! If you give me a son, I promise that I will dedicate him to you for his whole life . . . (1 Samuel 1:11).

Steps of Faith

When we reach this point there are two indispensable steps of faith we can take to get us back on the right track. The first is to *admit to ourselves, to our partner, and to God that we are ultimately powerless over our infertility and that our lives have become unmanageable because of this crisis.* This doesn't mean that there is nothing we can do to help ourselves. On the contrary, there is much we can choose to do. We can avail ourselves of the best medical treatment. We can join support groups or get therapy. What we cannot do is *will* ourselves into pregnancy and parenthood. Conception depends on too many variables over which we have no control. This is something we simply have to recognize and accept as a fact of life. The longer we fight against it the more out of control our lives become. Admitting our powerlessness opens the way for us to humbly ask God for the strength to face this crisis and to carry out His will for our lives.

This brings us to the second step. Next, we need to *make a daily, conscious, willful decision to turn our lives over to the care of God* as we understand God through Jesus Christ. Most of us feel we did that a long time ago, and maybe we did. But that was then. This is now. If we look closely at how we've been handling our struggle with infertility, we may be surprised at just how controlling, even manipulative, we have become. Some people, it seems, will stop at nothing to get a child. Others, like Hannah, bargain with God, promising to do this or that in exchange for a child.

These are examples of our trying to regain control over our destiny, to wrestle with God, refusing to let Him go unless He grants our wish. If we stop and think about it, we'll realize how this kind of behavior is exactly the opposite of the Christian attitude of humble servanthood. Deciding to turn our will and our lives over to God's care through Jesus Christ enables God once again to occupy that vital center of our lives, to give us an attitude of humility and the ability to trust Him to be with us through these difficult days.

When we take these two simple-sounding—but really quite difficult—steps of faith, we open our hearts and lives to the hope of God as never before.

Looking again at that passage from Ephesians, we discover the comforting promise of God's grace that will see us through to the resolution of our infertility crisis—be it conception, adoption, or childlessness.

As we said earlier, these verses reveal God's great hope for each of our lives: that we may "become mature people, reaching to the very height of Christ's full stature," and that we will "grow up in every way to Christ, who is the head." If we cooperate with God's grace by daily placing our lives, our wills, and our gifts into his hands, then, as Paul later wrote to the Philippians, we have the assurance that "God, who began this good work in you, will carry it on until it is finished on the Day of Christ Jesus" (Philippians 1:6).

Put another way, we have the assurance that if we will but remain faithful, God's grace will not ultimately be denied. Regardless of the particular outcome of our situation, God through Jesus Christ will keep working with our lives until He brings us, fully and completely, to the newness of life that broke forth into the world that first Easter Sunday.

THINGS TO DO

1. Admit to yourself, to God, and to your partner that you are powerless over your infertility. Understand that this does not necessarily mean you should stop treatment or give up in despair. By taking this step, you are acknowledging your finitude, your limits as a person, and that you cannot will or manipulate your way into parenthood.

2. Each morning, before you even get out of bed, make a conscious, prayerful decision to turn your will over to the care of God through Jesus Christ.

3. Determine that you will live this day to its fullest, responding to your own needs and those of others who may cross your path. Remember that this day is all that really counts, because none of us can live more than one day at a time.

By regaining a biblical perspective, you can discover a sense of hope, of meaning, of assurance, that is not dependent upon the outcome of your crisis.

6
Gaining Strength and Comfort from God's Word

WHETHER we conceive a child of our own, adopt, or remain childless, we have a unique role to play in God's eternal plan. As Paul wrote to the Ephesians:

Under *his control* all the different parts of the body fit together by every joint with which it is provided. So when each separate part works as it should, the whole body grows and builds itself up through love (Ephesians 4:16).

In other words, you have a special place of ministry, a purpose for your life that cannot be taken away by this illness. There is in Christ's church a place of service, of meaning, reserved for you. God's hope for you is that by turning your life and will over to Jesus Christ, you will find that unique place of service and continue to grow toward the fullness of life so clearly revealed in His Son.

Alan

Eventually the day came when I realized my vocation, my calling in life, was not going to change. Whether Patricia and I had one child, none, or ten, I was going to finish my doctorate, preach, do therapy, write, and publish. Either with children or without, we would continue to build a life together. Parenthood, I realized, was not the only path to personal fulfillment. Getting to this point of self-realization brought a certain sense of liberation, a recovery of the future—a future that would still be waiting regardless of the way our infertility situation was resolved. Regaining a biblical perspective is, in effect, a way of learning how to move from shock and denial, through treatment, and toward resolution without kicking, screaming, and fighting for control every step of the way.

Please don't misunderstand. We are not suggesting that you give up, stop treatment, sit back, and let happen whatever will. You need to avail yourself of the best medical, emotional, and spiritual resources you can find. We are suggesting that by regaining a biblical perspective, you can discover a sense of hope, of meaning, of assurance, that is *not* dependent upon the outcome of your crisis.

Turning to Scripture for Help

In Paul's letter to the church in Rome we find these words:

> We know that in all things God works for good with those who love him, those whom he has called according to his purpose (Romans 8:28).

Paul wasn't implying that God is the cause behind everything that happens to us. His faith had developed well beyond such simplistic assumptions. What he was saying was that there is no situation, no matter how hopeless it may look, no matter how painful it may become, where God cannot prevail and bring some good out of it.

This is true when applied to the infertility crisis as well. Even if you never conceive or adopt, you still have the possibility of growing through the crisis to ever deepening levels of faith, hope, and understanding. While such perseverance is difficult and often painful, Scripture can become for us a source of strength unlike any other, assuring us of God's unwavering love and helping us deal with our emotional chaos.

One couple we know, Terry and Denise, came up to me at a denominational meeting and asked if we might speak privately. They had heard Patricia and I were writing this book and wanted to share some of their experience with the hope it might help someone else.

About a year earlier they had reached the point where nothing else could be done; they had to either adopt or choose to remain childless. Both were in full-time Christian service. Denise told me how she had gone through a period when Scripture seemed to lose all its meaning. It was, she said, as if all these words were addressed to someone else. Then one day the thought came to her that these words of Paul were not intended for some abstract notion of humanity; they were God's special words to her, *personally*. She copied Romans 8:28 in large letters and posted them on their refrigerator door. She repeated them throughout the day, especially when she felt as though she had nothing to look forward to now that she knew she couldn't have a child.

"There are times," Terry said, "when we need to remember God is speaking directly *to us* in Scripture, and hang on to that because sometimes it's the only thing we have to hold on to." Wise advice.

Scripture speaks little of prolonged cases of infertility, and even less of sterility. Nevertheless, the biblical writers were familiar with all the emotions experienced by infertile couples. For example, Psalm 13 says:

> How much longer will you forget me, Lord? Forever? How much longer will you hide yourself from me? How long must I endure trouble? How long will sorrow fill my heart day and night? Look at me, O Lord my God, and answer me. Restore my strength; don't let me die.

The psalmist has expressed our feelings of abandonment, the fatigue that comes from struggling long and hard with difficult circumstances, and the painful grief of a life's desire left unfulfilled.

Dave and Brenda, whose story you will read in more detail in the next chapter, talked about this feeling of being abandoned by God. Dave had read the Psalms before, but he had never been in a situation where he could so readily identify with what the psalmist was feeling.

"The thing that struck me the hardest," he said, "was the way the writers of the Psalms still believed, still trusted even when they didn't feel anything of God's presence in their lives. I guess that's when faith really becomes faith; when we are faced with the choice of believing or not believing, trusting or not trusting, regardless of how we may feel at the moment."

In addition to the psalms that speak to our feelings are those that give us strength by encouraging trust in God's providential care. These verses from Psalm 46 have often spoken to my heart:

> God is our shelter and strength, always ready to help in times of trouble. So we will not be afraid, even if the earth is shaken and mountains fall into the ocean depths; even if the seas roar and rage, and the hills are shaken by the violence.

Other psalms dealing with themes of suffering, comfort, and strength in adversity are: Psalms 25, 27, 31, 42, 51, 63, 123, 130, and 139.

You may find other particularly meaningful Old Testament passages that deal with themes of hope and God's promise of deliverance to a beleaguered people. One of my favorites has always been these verses from Isaiah 40:

> Israel, why then do you complain that the Lord doesn't know your troubles or care if you suffer injustice? Don't you know? Haven't you heard? The Lord is the everlasting God; he created all the world. He never grows tired or weary. No one understands his thoughts. He strengthens those who are weak and tired. Even those who are young grow weak; young men can fall exhausted. But those who trust in the Lord for help will find their strength renewed. They will rise on wings like eagles; they will run and not get weary; they will walk and not grow weak (Isaiah 40:27–31).

Turning to the New Testament we find the words of Jesus: "Happy are those who mourn; God will comfort them!" (Matthew 5:4). And these words of promise:

> Come to me, all of you who are tired from carrying heavy loads, and I will give you rest. Take my yoke and

put it on you, and learn of me, because I am gentle and humble in spirit; and you will find rest. For the yoke I will give you is easy, and the load I will put on you is light (Matthew 11:28–30).

And in John's Gospel we find this:

I have told you this so that you will have peace by being united to me. The world will make you suffer. But be brave! I have defeated the world! (John 16:33)

The writings of Paul—who was himself well acquainted with physical, emotional, and spiritual anguish—assure us that no predicament, no matter how painful, can ever separate us from God's love.

For I am certain that nothing can separate us from his love: neither death nor life, neither angels nor other heavenly rulers or powers, neither the present nor the future, neither the world above nor the world below— there is nothing in all creation that will ever be able to separate us from the love of God which is ours through Christ Jesus our Lord (Romans 8:38,39).

As we read these and other helpful passages, it's important to remember that those who wrote the words were every bit as human as we are. They sensed the same hurt, were troubled by many of the same thoughts, felt overwhelmed under the burdens of struggles much like ours. Still, they prayed when they didn't feel like it. They trusted God when it looked as though every reason to trust had vanished, because faith sometimes means trusting even when you are emotionally, spiritually, and physically drained and hurting. By such discipline they learned the virtues of patience until patience finally gave way to renewed hope. The various circumstances they faced did not always turn out the way they wished. Yet each found the strength to endure their difficult times.

What About Healing?

One of the most difficult things we have to face as infertile couples is that the Gospels are full of accounts of Jesus healing a multitude of physical infirmities. Yet despite our ardent prayers, we still may not conceive. It's only natural to wonder why.

In Matthew's Gospel we read of Jesus healing a woman who had suffered for years from a painful menstrual disorder. She merely touches the hem of His garment and is suddenly healed. Jesus turns to her and says, "Courage, my daughter! Your faith has made you well" (Matthew 9:22).

Could it be, after all, that we have some spiritual deficiency, some lack of faith that makes it impossible for Christ to heal us? Are we to blame?

We do not believe you can blame yourselves for being infertile. Nor do we think you should chastise yourselves for not having enough faith when conception does not occur. Nowhere does Scripture promise physical healing to everyone who asks for it. True, healing does occur, sometimes miraculously. Many infertile couples conceive after having exhausted all relevant possibilities for medical treatment. And God also uses the wonders of medical science as extensions of His healing hands. Nonetheless, there are many couples who, despite fervent prayer and much faith, remain childless until they have sought adoption.

People of outstanding faith have often prayed for deliverance from physical ailments, even great pain, only to discover healing was not forthcoming. The apostle Paul, certainly a hero of faith, is one example.

In 2 Corinthians Paul writes of his own "painful physical ailment," from which he prayed three times to be delivered (2 Corinthians 12:7–10). Despite Paul's great faith and passionate belief in the power of prayer, no healing came.

Why? Perhaps part of the reason is that the world we live in is still not the Kingdom of God. The world, and those of us who live in it, is yet imperfect. God has not finished with creation, so it is still a place where joy mingles with sorrow, where the body and mind remain plagued by diseases, and where each of us must face death while clinging to the hope God gives for resurrection. Infertility, then, is a handicap that we must sometimes learn to cope with as best we can.

Can we take any comfort from those passages that recount Jesus' healings? Yes, if we interpret them properly.

First, we must remember that healing may yet come. Unless we have passed the age where childbearing is possible, there is still a chance for conception. Those for whom there remains even a slim chance should not give up hope that they may be one of those fortunate couples who conceive late in life, even after the treatment process has run its course and the possibility seems eliminated.

Second, we can view the healings of Jesus as promises that God will indeed complete the good work begun in each of us. When we look again at Ephesians 4:13—"we shall become mature people, reaching to the very height of Christ's full stature"—in light of Jesus' ministry of healing, we can reasonably conclude that God's hope for us includes physical healing. What Paul means by *maturity* may be understood as physical health, and spiritual and emotional well-being. Jesus' healings are signs of God's power. They point us ahead to the day when God's Kingdom will be established among us. On that day God will have finally overcome every form of physical impairment, emotional pain, even death itself. But for now we must live in and cope with the world we have.

So if there is no certainty of physical healing now, what then can we hope for? We can hope and pray for the healing of our emotions, for the binding up of broken dreams, for the mending and strengthening of marriages too long burdened with childlessness and its cycles of hope and depression. We can hope for Christ's healing presence as we work through our grief, knowing that God understands and is well acquainted with our sorrow. We can pray for our self-image, knowing that through persistent faith we can once again piece together our shattered self-esteem. Physical healing may or may not come, but emotional and spiritual healing must come if we are to grow through the infertility crisis to become effective participants in Christ's reconciling work.

Indeed, emotional and spiritual healing must be attended to regardless of the outcome of the immediate crisis. The psychological scars of the grief, and the wounds the stress may have inflicted upon our relationships, are not automatically healed even with conception and the birth of a healthy child. Unless we address any areas of our lives where infertility has left emotional scar tissue, our self-esteem, and maybe even our marriage, may never fully recover. We must bring all these issues, sometimes with the aid of a trained therapist and a minister who understands, before the altar of God's healing grace.

Whether you conceive, adopt, or remain childless, you will find the healing grace that enables you to continue faith's journey. The apostle Paul found that despite his physical affliction, God's grace provided strength enough to help him grow through his crisis. God promises to do the same for you.

THINGS TO DO

1. Carefully read each Scripture mentioned in this chapter.

2. Try to get in touch with what the writer is feeling, especially the writers of the Psalms.

3. Identify your own feelings. Find those Scripture passages that most accurately reflect them.

4. Note how the biblical writer deals with the situation, how the writer manages to trust even though God seems far removed from his or her presence.

5. Begin reading Scripture as God's Word addressed directly to you in your specific situation.

6. Realize that this is one of those times when faith becomes a matter of your will rather than your emotions. Know that you can choose to trust even when you don't feel like trusting.

7. Know that God has not given up, that He is even now aware of your predicament, working to bring good out of it even when you can't see how that could possibly be true.

There are times when we feel God
has walked out on us.

7
Where Are You, God?

Alan

BRENDA sat on my office couch, hands in her lap, slowly grinding into small bits the tissue she'd been using to wipe away her tears. Dave, her husband of seven years, sat with his arm around her. Theirs was a difficult situation. Brenda had undergone surgery to repair blocked fallopian tubes, while Dave had been receiving treatment for a low sperm count.

"You remember when Brenda had her surgery last year," he began. "Well, we thought unblocking the fallopian tubes would do it—that, combined with my treatments and the fertility drugs. But nothing has happened and it's been a year."

Brenda interrupted. "It's just getting worse. Every month we get our hopes up, then nothing happens. I've tried to be positive but it's getting harder all the time. Sometimes I get so depressed. I don't want to go to work, and when I'm there it's hard to concentrate. There's a lady in our office who's six months pregnant. I passed her in the hall last week and it was all I could do to keep from crying."

"I know this ordeal has put a great deal of stress on both of you and on your marriage," I said. "And believe me, I do understand the depression and frustration you're feeling. But if I'm really going to help you I need to hear from both of you. Dave, what about you?"

"Well, it's like you said, frustrating. I just get angry," Dave said. "Here we are doing everything we're supposed to be doing. But what good is it? I hate the feeling of being up against something I've got no control over.

"I hate seeing her go through this. I can't stand not being able to do anything. And I really *can't*. I get so angry. Sometimes I just want to yell and scream at somebody, hit something."

"Are you angry with Brenda?"

"Of course not. She can't help it. I guess I'm angry because none of this makes any sense."

"What doesn't make sense?"

"The whole infertility thing. I mean, why is this happening? You know as well as I that there are hundreds, maybe even thousands of abortions every day in this country. There was even a story in the paper the other day about a teenager who dumped her newborn into a trash can because she didn't want her parents to know she was pregnant—though heaven only knows how she managed to hide it for nine months. And here we are—we've got a nice home, good careers. We're Christians. And Brenda's right; we've prayed so much that I'm beginning to think it's useless. I don't want to offend you, Alan. But if there really is a God, well, either He doesn't care enough to do anything, or maybe He can't. It probably isn't right to feel that way, but I can't help it."

"I understand what you're saying, Dave. And there's absolutely nothing wrong with what you're feeling and thinking. You have a right to be angry. It's not fair that a couple with as much to offer a child as the two of you can't have one. It isn't fair, and it's wrong when frightened teen-agers dump infants into trash cans or get abortions while Brenda spends a week in the hospital and you run back and forth to the doctor's office twice a month. There are times—this is certainly one of them—when we feel God has walked out on us. After what the two of you have been through, I'd be surprised if you weren't feeling all this. What about you, Brenda? Do you feel the same way?"

"Not exactly," she said, without looking up. "But it's different for me, I guess. I'm the one who's cursed or broken or whatever else you want to call it."

"What do you mean, 'cursed'? Sounds to me like you think God is out to get you."

"I guess maybe He is," she said. "I was pretty wild back when I was in school. I don't mean that I was promiscuous or anything like that; just that I was never much of a can-didate for sainthood. Maybe it's all catching up with me. Doesn't the Bible talk about your sins finding you out or coming back to haunt you or something like that?"

"Are you saying you think God is punishing you by keeping you from having a baby?"

"It's possible, isn't it? At least that's what it feels like. I've always thought I'd make a good mother, and I know Dave would make a great father. But maybe I wouldn't; maybe God knows I'd make a terrible mother, too demanding. Maybe I just don't deserve a baby.

"Like Dave said, we've prayed about this a lot. I've promised God I'd change if He'd just let me know what's wrong about me—about us—that He wants changed. Who knows? If I hadn't done that stuff back in school, or if I weren't such a perfectionist, or didn't want both a career and a baby, maybe then 'God would find favor with me' like it says in the Bible."

Every couple's struggle with infertility is somewhat different, but my conversation with Dave and Brenda revealed many of the faith questions that infertile couples often wrestle with. Dave's anger and frustration are understandable. It's natural to be angry when you are hurting. And he's right about infertility not being fair. But beneath his anger and frustration he's beginning to grapple with questions as old as the Book of Job. Why is this happening? How can he continue believing in a God of compassionate love when abortions take place every day, children are abused or abandoned, while he and Brenda remain childless?

Brenda is wondering whether her current inability to conceive is God's punishment for some things she did in her past. She feels "cursed" or "broken," that something is defective with her *as a person*. Depressed and exhausted, she's questioning whether she even deserves to be a mother because she thinks she would be a parental failure.

Both are struggling with the usefulness of prayer. What good is it when our prayers aren't being answered? Why doesn't God do something? Why doesn't He help? Can't He see our suffering, our pain? Where is God in all this anyway? How can we go on believing when our faith has hit a brick wall?

Let's take these three basic issues and deal with them individually.

Infertility Is Unfair

We all know life is unfair. Bad things happen to good people. Most of us don't have any trouble accepting that fact—until life doesn't play fair with *us*. Then, like Dave, we begin questioning the goodness of God—we may even doubt whether there is a God. But can we really blame God for infertility, for life's unfairness? Or does the problem lie elsewhere?

I believe God creates each of us with a certain amount of freedom. And most of the injustices we see around us result from the abuse of that freedom. We can't, for example, blame God for the abortion problem because God isn't responsible for illegitimate or unwanted pregnancy. Neither can we blame God for child abuse since God isn't the one entrusted with the responsibility of raising a child. At times we all abuse our God-given freedom. This doesn't mean freedom is a bad thing. It simply means that we have the capacity to make good or bad decisions. And every decision we make has its consequences.

Dave is right. Their infertility isn't fair. But the unfairness isn't due to God's malevolence. God gives us freedom because He wants each of us to have a choice in how we live and how—or whether—we will relate to our Creator. Without freedom we would lack the capacity to form relationships either with God or with one another.

Still, an even more difficult question lurks just below the surface: the question of disability and disease. How can Dave and Brenda continue believing in God's compassionate love in the midst of their suffering? Are we to believe that God causes not only infertility, but such things as cancer, birth defects, and all sorts of other debilitating maladies? And what about those infertile women in the Bible who, as we have seen in an earlier chapter, clearly felt that God was at the heart of their difficulties? Doesn't that indicate God is somehow the cause of all this?

First, we need to remember that in biblical times people did not share our modern understanding of the human body. For Rachel, Sarah, and the others, either God or evil spirits were the cause of everything. But through modern medical science we have come to know how sickness can be brought on through infections, and how disabilities can arise from malfunctions of our biological systems.

Personally, we do not believe God is responsible for infertility or cancer any more than we can say God is responsible for tornados or earthquakes. There is a certain randomness, an element of chance, built into the very structure of the universe. If you have been in treatment very long, I'm sure your doctor has already explained how many factors could contribute to your current inability to bear a child. Our reproductive systems are complex. Successful conception involves a long process of biological events. Like pieces in a jigsaw puzzle, each has to fall into place at just the right moment to get the desired result. If even one thing goes wrong along the way, our reproductive process may be in trouble.

Is this any way to run a universe? Couldn't God have invented a world where nothing ever goes wrong, where no one ever gets sick, and every child is born in perfect health? These questions, legitimate though they are, lead well beyond the scope of this book. We would encourage you to pursue them if that is your desire, but at this point we must recognize that we have to deal with the world as we find it and move on.

Infertility and other physical problems are facts of life. But to say something is a fact of life isn't the same as saying God is responsible for it. Rather, it is a way of affirming what we instinctively know: that God has created a world in which there is a chance of things going wrong. Reproductive systems may malfunction or be damaged by illnesses like appendicitis, or we may be injured in an accident. Any number of factors may result in infertility, but we honestly do not believe God is one of them.

As we learned in Chapter 5, God's will is for every couple who desires a child to have one. Yet even God's will can sometimes be thwarted by adverse circumstances.

Am I Being Punished for Something?

Brenda wonders whether God is punishing her because of her past. She wonders if she would turn out to be a terrible mother. Her self-esteem is taking a beating because she's sure that somehow the infertility is her fault.

None of us is without sin, of course. Dave could well be wondering the same thing. Maybe the problem lies hidden somewhere in his past. Perhaps all this is his fault. Although he hasn't said it in so many words, Dave may be getting ready to accompany Brenda on her guilt trip.

This is natural. But even though most infertile couples wonder if it isn't somehow their fault, the only thing faulty is the thinking. And the danger is, if we don't get our thinking straight, we will begin the downward spiral through guilt into the bottomless pit of depression.

It's true that we do bear the consequences of our behavior. When we do something wrong we feel guilty. When it's legitimate, guilt is God's way of letting us know that we need to make some changes in our lives. It's a sign that we need to ask God's forgiveness, and, where necessary, the forgiveness of others so we can get on with our lives.

At this point we need to reaffirm the central tenet of our Christian faith: that Jesus Christ took the burden of our sins upon Himself so that we might experience God's forgiveness and find new life. God does not want us to beat ourselves into the ground and ruin our lives and the lives of those close to us by continuing to carry the weight of our sinful past. The Good News of God in Christ is that our past sins, whatever they may be, are not held against us.

But what if, as a result of past behavior, you contracted a Sexually Transmitted Disease (STD) that is contributing to your inability to conceive? Does that mean your infertility is God's punishment?

Here we need to distinguish between consequence and punishment. STDs can contribute to infertility, but they are consequences of our actions and those of others. They are not God's way of getting back at infertile couples who have—like everyone else—sinned and fallen short of God's glory.

Hannah, whose story we find in 1 Samuel 1–2, is a good biblical example for infertile couples. In great misery, Hannah "poured out her troubles to the Lord" (1 Samuel 1:15). Whether the feelings are anxiety over the future, or guilt, or doubts about our ability to parent, from time to time we all need to "pour out our troubles to the Lord," to confess our sins and ask forgiveness, and to surrender our predicament into God's caring hands.

It's well known that the kind of severe emotional and physical stress Brenda and Dave are experiencing is sometimes a deterrent to pregnancy—though this is rarely the sole cause of infertility. Occasionally an infertile couple adopts a child, then a few months or years later the wife becomes pregnant. The deciding factor in such cases may be *surrender.* Giving up their struggle, they relax and determine to get on with their lives. The quest for pregnancy no longer dominates the stage.

Dave and Brenda, like so many infertile couples, have let their desire for a child become an obsession. It occupies center stage in their lives, a place only God in Christ can fill. Surrender, confession, and forgiveness—pleading our case and leaving it on God's altar—leads to a new freedom from the anxieties that oppress us by restoring Christ to His rightful place. Sometimes this emotional release aids the reproductive process just enough. But unless Brenda and Dave, like Hannah, are willing to "pour out their troubles to the Lord," they may never know.

Concerns about their future ability to parent are likewise unfounded. Their doubts stem primarily from the drubbing their self-esteem is taking, their feelings of failure as a man and a woman, the emotional and physical exhaustion of the treatment process. With Brenda and Dave's dedication to their Christian faith, their commitment to each other and their willingness to grow as a couple, there is no reason to believe they wouldn't be fine parents. Not perfect, mind you, but good enough.

Besides, we can look around us and see God doesn't grant children based on the ability to be a successful parent. Were that the case, there would be no such thing as child abuse.

God is punishing neither Dave nor Brenda. Dave and Brenda are punishing themselves by refusing to surrender their situation to Jesus Christ, who alone has rightful claim to center stage.

Where Are You, God?

Much of Dave and Brenda's anxiety stems from feeling their prayers go no higher than the ceiling. They each have experienced what the psalmist felt when he wrote:

> My God, my God, why have you abandoned me? I have cried desperately for help, but still it does not come. During the day I call to you, my God, but you do not answer; I call at night, but get no rest (Psalm 22:1,2).

Under stressful circumstances our prayers often become a desperate search for God's presence in the midst of suffering, an impassioned plea for a miracle or a way of trying to bargain with God. Dave and Brenda asked for a miracle. Offering to make whatever changes God wanted, they bargained. Still, nothing has happened. Now they are beginning to face the possibility that they may never bear their own child.

Psalm 22 is a lament, the prayer of a man in desperate circumstances, a man who feels despised, rejected, completely overwhelmed by his troubles. Yet he is still willing to let God occupy the center of his life. After pouring out his troubles before the Lord, he writes:

> I will tell my people what you have done; I will praise you in their assembly: "Praise him, you servants of the Lord! Honor him, you descendants of Jacob! Worship him, you people of Israel!" (Psalm 22:22,23)

Here is the prayer of a man who, though in great emotional pain, has learned not only to trust but also even to praise God in those troubled times.

As painful as it may be for them, Brenda and Dave need to realize that God never promised to wave a magic wand and make all our troubles fade away. True, miracles still happen. Sometimes. And while it's too soon for them to give up their quest to conceive, it isn't too early to begin to understand that for some couples the miracle they prayed for just never comes. But, as the writer of Psalm 22 discovered, this does not mean God has abandoned them.

What God promises is the gift of His presence. "If you love me, you will obey my commandments," Jesus said. "And I will ask the Father, and he will give you another Helper, who will stay with you forever . . . When I go, you will not be left alone; I will come back to you" (John 14:15,16,18).

In these few sentences we find Jesus' prescription for getting through those disillusioning days when we're struggling with the frightening possibility that we may never bear our own child.

We begin by trusting that God loves us and wants the best for us. We realize that our present circumstances stem from living in an imperfect world where people get sick and suffer all sorts of tragedy. And that our infertility is not a sign of God's vengeance or disfavor, no matter what we may have done in the past.

As best we can, we continue day by day with whatever work God has given us to do at this point in our lives. We continue in prayer and in regular worship and fellowship with other Christians because these are often the special people God chooses to comfort and care for us. Maintaining private devotion, we remain open to God's will, trusting God to reveal the next steps for us to take when the time— God's time—is right.

These are the disciplines of the spiritual life that are the essence of obedience. And in response to our obedience the Spirit, Helper, Comforter, Healer of life's wounds, comes into our hearts and lives. Grieved though we may be, fearing childlessness, uncertain about the adoption that may or may not lie in our future, in that all-embracing Presence we discover God's own assurance that we have not been and will not be abandoned.

Conclusion

The God who reveals Himself to us in Jesus Christ does not hold our sins against us. He offers us instead His gracious forgiveness, releasing us from burdens of guilt that we no longer need to carry. Infertility is not God's punishment. Rather, like so many other maladies of the human condition, it is a handicap caused by malfunctions of our bodies' reproductive system. And though God has not promised to always work miracles on our behalf, we can take comfort in Jesus' assurance that we do not bear the burdens of infertility alone. Through God's presence with us in the power of the Holy Spirit, we discover the strength we need to either suspend treatment and remain childless, or choose to pursue adoption.

THINGS TO DO

1. Take a sheet of paper and write down all the problems, doubts, uncertainties, etc., about your relationship with God that you have had since beginning your struggle with infertility.

2. Examine them in light of what we have discussed in these last three chapters.

3. Decide whether there are outmoded beliefs or immature ways of thinking about God that you might need to get rid of. Recognize that it's okay to jettison outmoded ways of believing and thinking, since this is part of our growth process as Christians.

4. Make a list of the ways your thinking about God has changed, now that you have read these last three chapters.

5. If your faith is still "shaky," go to your minister or another trained therapist and discuss these faith issues thoroughly. Keep working through your doubts until you come to the place where your faith is renewed through deeper understanding.

When the distinction between the desire to conceive and the call to parenthood is clear, then you may be ready to consider one of the many adoption alternatives.

8
Should We Adopt?

Alan

PARENTING is a vocation. Conception, pregnancy, and birth are physical experiences that lead to our assuming the role of parents. Sometimes the distinction gets lost in an obsessive desire of many infertile couples to conceive and give birth.

You want the pregnancy experience, and you are frustrated, hurt, and angry when it seems as though the vicissitudes of life are robbing you of that blessed event. Your grief becomes more intense as you near the end of your treatment options. You may have thought briefly of adoption in the past, but now it looms ahead as a real possibility, even a necessity if you are ever to have a child of your own.

At this point you need to examine more deeply your motives. Are you thinking of adoption as "the next best thing to pregnancy"? Are you approaching it with the idea that once you adopt you might later conceive "a child of your own"? If these are your thoughts, then we suggest you are not ready to become adoptive parents.

An adopted child is neither second best nor a means to post-adoptive pregnancy. Both of you must be willing to accept, love, and care for an adopted child in exactly the same way as you would a baby naturally conceived. So ask yourselves this: If you adopt now and get pregnant later, would there be any difference in your feelings for your adopted child? Could you love *both* equally, without distinction?

The question is of utmost importance, but it's not an easy one to answer. Patricia was ready to try adoption much sooner than I was. I remember struggling for months over whether I could truly love a child that wasn't mine in the traditional sense.

How you answer that question depends on your under-standing of the word *mine.* By mine we usually mean a child born by means of our own natural biological proces-ses, a child with whom we are physically bonded through the miracle of conception.

Though the biological bond between parent and child is one way of being connected, there are others even more important. Emotional bonds of love, care, and friendship can, and indeed must, form over time between parent and child. These *relational* ties we build with our child make us *parents.* Without them it matters little whether we are the "real" father or "real" mother. When I finally realized the biological link was secondary to the relationship, I knew I was as ready as Patricia to begin the adoption process.

If you want a child to love, raise, teach, and care for, a child who will return your love as you move through life, then you are beginning to understand what parenting is all about. When parenting is your vocation, your calling in life, then the particular *way* a child comes into your family is not your main concern.

When the distinction between the desire to conceive and the call to parenthood is clear, then you too may be ready to consider one of the many adoption alternatives. The question, "Can I really love a child that isn't mine," is understood in a very different light. A child becomes "ours" through the parental relationship of mutual love and caring, through the psychological and spiritual bonding that runs far deeper than any biological connection ever could.

Besides, our children are never really "ours." They are not possessions we own like so much furniture. Whether they come to us through adoption or conception, they are God's children. As parents we are stewards of their lives. God has entrusted them, like everything else in life, to our care. Adoption becomes an option when we find ourselves wanting to accept this most sacred trust.

When to Begin

One of the most difficult decisions facing infertile couples is when to begin the adoption process. Two things, the practice of abortion and the trend toward more teenage mothers keeping their babies, mean there are fewer children available to prospective parents. Waiting periods between application and placement may be from three to six years or more. Couples often ask, "Do we start proceedings now, while still in treatment, or wait until we've exhausted all possibilities of conceiving our own?"

Several factors are important here, and each must be weighed carefully in light of your individual circumstances. Age is crucial. If you and your spouse have waited to start a family, you may be coming close to the cutoff date after which many adoption agencies will no longer accept you as parental candidates. While various agencies do differ, many will not accept applicants over age 35 or so.

Where you are in the treatment process, the options remaining open, and the odds your specialist gives you of succeeding are also critical. At this point your doctor needs to be perfectly honest with you about your chances. If you are running out of time and alternatives, it may be best to begin now. Should you get pregnant you can always call the agency and withdraw your application. The agency will be delighted for you and happy they can now provide a child to another anxious couple.

Be aware that some adoption agencies require either group or individual counseling. Even if they don't, counseling is a good idea. You need to be sure parenting is your true motivation. You need to deal with the grief of knowing you probably will never conceive and give birth, and to begin working through the many alternatives that adoption opens to you.

Adoption: Sorting Out the Options

After deciding to pursue adoption, we contacted a local church-affiliated agency to begin the application process. We attended an inquiry meeting for prospective parents, and were surprised that more than thirty other couples were there. The placement specialist introduced us to many options we had never before considered.

Like most of the other couples, we are Caucasian, and our first preference was for a white infant. We quickly learned that the demand is highest for Caucasian newborns, which means there are fewer available. If we were committed to considering only an infant of the same racial heritage as ours, we could count on at least a six-year wait.

A Child of Another Race?

We were confronted with the first major decision every couple faces. Do we want a child of our same race? Or would we consider adopting a child with a different ethnic, racial, or cultural background?

Adopting across racial and ethnic lines calls for special consideration. It's sad to say, but a good deal of prejudice still exists. Prejudice is learned behavior, and when thinking about it, you may encounter remnants of prejudice that were ingrained in you during childhood. Confronting your own prejudices may make you uncomfortable, even ashamed, for having second thoughts about adopting a child of another race. But this is the time for brutal honesty —with yourself, your spouse, and your extended family.

Fortunately, with God's help we can overcome our latent prejudices. Many couples quite successfully adopt children of different backgrounds. Those who do so provide an abiding witness to their faith in the colorblind God who creates all children, be they "red or yellow, black or white," in God's own image.

Other aspects of cross-cultural adoptions are equally important. It takes special care to explain to a child why he or she is of a different color or has physical characteristics that are different from the parents'. And while you may have no trouble accepting such a child into your home, your relatives may not have the same openness. Will your child be accepted by his or her grandparents, cousins, aunts, and uncles? If not, there is the potential for conflict within your extended family, which can put a great strain on your marriage and the parent/child relationship. If you have any doubts, it's better to ask your relatives how they feel before you proceed, then prepare yourselves for the consequences of your decision.

There is also the question of how you, yourselves, will relate to your child's racial and cultural heritage. African-American children raised by white parents, and vice versa, may find themselves caught between cultures, especially during the identity-forming years of adolescence. Are you prepared to raise your child as heir to *both* cultures, affirming the contributions of each? Will you let your child freely choose the culture he or she will identify with the most? Or will you try to pour your child into your own racial/cultural mold?

Due to these issues, some agencies will not allow cross-racial adoptions—but others will. Still others decide on a case-by-case basis. Some even specialize in these types of adoptions, providing counseling and follow-up help for the new family. Whatever you decide, it's best to be clear and up-front with the agencies about your intentions.

It takes special people, people of deep faith and great courage, to adopt across racial, ethnic, and cultural boundaries. On the other hand, you need not feel guilty if, after giving the subject prayerful thought, you decide you are not so inclined. This doesn't mean you are less a Christian than those who are. It just means that as prospective parents you may not be suited to the special demands of this particular highly challenging role.

An Older Child?

If you don't want to wait for an infant or decide you are not good prospects for cross-racial adoption, you may want to consider adopting an older child. Since demand is greatest for newborns, waiting lists for older children are usually shorter. But this too is a very special calling.

Older children come with special needs that require unique parenting skills. Some may have been physically, even sexually, abused. Many have experienced emotional abuse. Often the older child carries deep wounds of rejection and feels unwanted, even unlovable. Not a few have been shuffled from foster home to foster home. Some have behavioral problems caused by living in an environment where proper nurturing was unavailable.

Older children need to learn how to trust, to receive love as well as how to give it. They need to rebuild their shattered self-esteem and overcome the guilt often associated with rejection. None of this happens quickly. You will need to be the kind of parent who doesn't panic when periods of good behavior are interspersed with temper tantrums or other undesirable behavior, such as stealing or long days of withdrawal. Above all you will need to maintain a faith that believes miracles happen, that even the most scarred lives may—with patience, courage and love—be turned around.

Unlike infant adoption, the older child may have brothers and sisters, even birth parents, with whom he or she may need to relate throughout the rest of their lives. For good or ill, this links your family with theirs for years to come.

Boy or Girl?
You also need to decide how important it is for you to have a boy or a girl, or whether it matters. You may have a preference, and some agencies allow you to choose. For

some couples it's extremely important to have a male who can carry on the family name. Our feeling is that if you truly want to be parents, the sex of the child doesn't matter. If a legacy is what you are concerned about, you need to realize that the most important things our children carry into future generations have little to do with family names.

Disabled Children?

One of the most difficult decisions is whether to consider a disabled child. Disabled children fall into two categories: those who will never get better, such as victims of cerebral palsy, severe retardation, or uncorrectable physical problems; and those who will get better if provided with a good family atmosphere and proper medical and/or psychological care.

First, you need to decide which category you would be most comfortable dealing with. Second, decide whether you are best suited to deal with emotional or physical disabilities, or perhaps a combination of both. Third, consider the extra financial costs involved. Can you remodel the house to make it wheelchair accessible? Can you afford medical expenses well beyond those of a healthy child? What about education? Are there special or public schools in your area with appropriate rehabilitation programs?

Should you decide you have the unique aptitude necessary for parenting a special-needs child, the extra costs might not be the deciding factor. Financial help may be available. In 1980, Congress passed the Federal Adoption Assistance and Child Welfare Act (PL 96-272), which encourages the adoption of disabled children by providing financial support to willing parents. Since the program is administered through the states, it may or may not be available in your area. Before you make a final decision, call your local child welfare office or adoption agency. They can tell you if federal funds are available, and whether you qualify.

After you have prayerfully, honestly considered the options and decided which are most appealing, then you are ready to move more fully into the adoption process.

Methods of Adoption

If you want to adopt, our advice is to explore every option. Because demand exceeds supply in just about every area, you must aggressively pursue every legal avenue.

First, contact the public welfare agency in your city or county. The Welfare Department handles adoptions, and since the agency is government supported, it is by far the least expensive. It is also where you will find the longest waiting list, especially for newborns. Contact them anyway, and get to know a case worker. This relationship will be very important since the laws of each state require an approved home study—which we will explain in greater detail a bit later—and most of these are handled through the Welfare Department. It is to your advantage to have a home study already approved as you begin pursuing other avenues.

Next, contact all the private adoption agencies in your area. Most private agencies are run by church and other charitable organizations. Some are self-supporting, professional agencies—with higher fees, of course. But many base fees on percentage of income with minimum and maximum limits.

Be sure to ask about any requirements. Some agencies, for example, prefer that the mother not work outside the home for the first three to five years. Certain levels of income and education may be required. And there are some who will not take your application if they know you are still pursuing infertility treatment. Upper and lower age limits may vary. Along with the agencies that specialize in cross-racial adoptions, some even handle international adoptions, while, as we said before, others forbid adoptions by parents of a different race or nationality. Religious agencies may prefer that applicants belong to their denomination or specific faith community. You may be asked to present documented evidence of your infertility. The important thing is to be clear about what you want and get on the waiting list as soon as you have made your decision.

To make sure you cover all the bases, I suggest you go to your local library and check out a copy of *The Child Welfare League of America's Guide to Adoption Agencies: A National Directory of Adoption Agencies and Adoption Resources*. If your library doesn't have one, request a copy from the following address:

> The Child Welfare League of America
> 440 First Street, North West, Suite 310
> Washington, D.C. 20001-2085

This is a state-by-state directory of both public and private agencies that explains their policies, lists fees and requirements and even the average waiting periods. There are more places to look than you may know about. The more contacts you make, the more you increase your chances of becoming adoptive parents.

Beyond public and private agencies, there is the option of independent adoption. Independent adoptions are usually handled through attorneys and physicians who know of a woman who wants to put her unborn child up for adoption but does not want to go through an agency.

The birth mother's reasons for not wanting to go the agency route may vary. She may want more control over the choice of parents than an agency would allow. She may want to specify race, geographical location, income and education levels, or whether the adoptive mother will work outside the home. In some instances, the birth mother may even insist on meeting prospective parents to decide for herself, or she may want to establish legal grounds for later contact with her child.

Independent adoptions are risky—and expensive. This doesn't mean you shouldn't pursue the option, though you must exercise more caution than is necessary when going through a long-established public or private agency. The birth mother may have had little or no counseling. Unsure of what she wants, she may change her mind at the last minute, leaving you emotionally and financially devastated. You may have no knowledge of the birth mother's health, which means your adopted child may suffer drug withdrawal or fetal alcohol syndrome. Little may be known about the birth mother's family background. And unless all the legal bases are covered, there is a slight chance that an independent adoption may be voided by the courts.

For these reasons, our advice is, *Hire your own attorney.* Make sure you are represented by legal counsel who is current on the adoption laws and procedures in your state. *Do not use an attorney provided by either the birth mother or her physician.* While the vast majority of doctors and lawyers dealing with independent adoptions are honest, caring persons, there are charlatans around who seek nothing but their own profit. If anyone involved refuses to deal with you unless you use his or her attorney, walk away. No reputable attorney or physician will object to your getting your own legal counsel. We cannot overemphasize how important this is. Should the court even suspect something is wrong, you stand a good chance of losing everything.

Due to the potential for illegality and fraud, independent adoptions are not permitted in some states. At this writing, they are illegal in Connecticut, Delaware, Massachusetts, Michigan, Minnesota, and North Dakota. The only way to make sure of the laws governing your state is to check with an attorney who is knowledgeable about current procedures.

Know beforehand that you will most likely have to pay all costs. This includes doctor bills for the birth mother's prenatal care and the delivery itself, hospital fees, counseling if she wants it, her attorney's costs as well as yours, plus court costs.

If you are willing to take the risks, you have the financial resources, and you have hired your own attorney, then leave no possibility unexplored. Have your lawyer contact others throughout the area. Get on the phone and contact obstetricians and general practitioners both in your town and in others nearby. You may even want to run ads in several newspapers (have respondents contact your attorney, not you). The more people who know you are looking, the more likely you are to find a birth mother considering allowing her baby to be adopted.

The Home Study

Every adoption—public, private, or independent—requires a home study, usually done by a local Welfare Department case worker. The very idea strikes terror into the heart of every potential parent. What is this person looking for? Is she going to open my drawers to check whether my socks are properly matched? Run her hand across the top of the china cabinet to see how often we dust?

Don't panic. A home study is done for one reason: to see if this is a home where a child will be provided with all he or she needs—physically, emotionally, and spiritually—to grow into a healthy adult. No one is turned down because there is dust on the coffee table.

Your case worker will write a report that will include a brief family history, your ages, income, your reasons for wanting to adopt, your plans for your child's education, how you plan to deal with the tremendous changes a child brings, infertility history and whether you are still in treatment, and so forth. If there are negatives in your past, such as your parents were divorced or you had an unhappy childhood, present them in a positive light. Show you have learned from your experiences and will provide better parenting than you received.

Granted, all this sounds like a tremendous intrusion into your privacy. And it is. But remember what's happening here. *You are asking the birth mother to give you her child.* Put yourself in her place. Wouldn't you want someone to make sure your child was being placed into the right hands?

Conclusion

Conception, pregnancy, and birth are biological processes. Parenting is a vocation, a sacred responsibility bestowed on us by our Creator. Once you have determined that your overarching desire is to parent, then you are ready to pursue one or several of the possible options offered by the adoption process.

THINGS TO DO

1. Now is the time to honestly evaluate, with your specialist's help, where you are in the process of infertility treatment. How old are you? How many more treatment options remain? Which ones might be feasible for you? Ask you doctor what he or she honestly thinks your odds are for conception.

2. Remember, even if you decide to continue treatment, nothing says you can't at least begin thinking about adoption. Go back over the options in this chapter, and prayerfully consider each. Discuss them with your spouse. Be honest with your feelings about such things as cross-cultural and cross-racial adoption.

3. Evaluate your financial status. Which options can you reasonably afford?

4. If you decide to begin the adoption process, start making the contacts we've suggested. Leave no stone unturned. The more doctors and agencies you contact, the more waiting lists you get on, the higher your chances of getting the child best suited for you.

Some infertility treatments raise difficult moral, ethical, and legal questions that must be dealt with openly before you proceed.

9

The Brave New World of Test-Tube Babies

MEDICAL science has been trying for years to solve the problems of infertility. But it was not until Louise Brown, the world's first "test-tube baby," was born on July 24, 1978, in Oldham, England, that words like *in vitro* fertilization became front-page news. Drs. Robert Edwards and Patrick Steptoe had done what many believed impossible: fertilized a human ovum in a glass dish and successfully transferred the embryo into the uterus where the normal development of pregnancy followed.

But from the midst of celebration there arose voices of concern. Science had begun to tinker with the very essence of life. The medical genie was out of the bottle and with him flew a host of moral and legal questions: Should doctors "play God"? Should the embryo be considered a "person," with all the legal rights and protections of the Constitution? Is discarding unused embryos the same as abortion? Would this technology usher in some sort of "brave new world" where conception would be separated from sexual intercourse and parental commitment?

These issues are far from settled. Fearing biological disaster, some feel medical technology has no business tampering with conception. Others believe just as passionately that whatever can be done should be done to help infertile couples.

This book is not a textbook on biomedical ethics. Examining all the intricate legal, moral, and theological questions involved in alternative reproductive technology would take many volumes. Our task here is simply to present an overview of the available options and point out some of the more obvious ethical considerations for you to think about. Please understand that we are not *recommending* any of these procedures. We simply want to introduce you to some of your options and raise some of the more basic questions you need to ask before proceeding with these treatments.

As you consider your options, we do, however, want to offer a word of caution. When in doubt about whether a particular treatment is right for you, we think it's always best to go along with the more conservative side of the moral question. Biomedical ethics presents us with a lot of moral gray areas where we cannot always be as sure of right and wrong as we would like to be. We have found that when one has serious doubts about undergoing a particular procedure it's always best to go with the more conservative position, at least until you have thought things through more thoroughly and come to a more decisive point in your decision-making process.

Again, it is not our place to recommend any of these alternative methods. Our task is merely to introduce you to the available medical technology and begin to raise the ethical questions you need to take into consideration before you proceed with any particular treatment.

God, Healing, and Modern Medicine

First we must set our discussion in the context of Scripture, the primary guide for all our moral decision-making.

In Chapter 5 we discussed how infertility is contrary to God's will. Infertility is a malfunction in the body's reproductive processes that prohibits our fulfilling God's command to "be fruitful and multiply" (Genesis 1:28).

The Bible gives us no specific rules to follow when it comes to making decisions about alternative reproductive methods like *in vitro* fertilization and embryo transfer. Such concerns were as far removed from the biblical world as space travel from the days of ox-drawn carts. We can, though, arrive at some basic biblical guidelines to help us sort out the complex moral issues in this brave new world of reproductive science.

We begin with our personal relationship with God through Jesus Christ. Based on our commitment to Him and openness to the leadership of His Spirit in our lives, we turn to Scripture for a better understanding of how we should live. We are yet sinful, and we will at times make wrong choices, but Christ expects us to use our God-given intelligence to make important decisions. So we forge ahead, taking the risks of faith and asking God's guidance on which options may be morally and medically best *for us*.

Healing is a basic theme in both Old and New Testaments. Prophets healed people in the name of a God of loving compassion. The Gospels are replete with examples of Jesus healing the sick and even raising the dead. When people suffer from infirmities, God often acts through human agents to restore them to health. This tells us that God's ideal is for us to be well, to be whole in body, mind, and spirit.

Next, nothing in either the Old or New Testament prohibits the use of medical treatment. There have always been doctors who used their various homemade remedies to heal the sick. Jesus mentions physicians, quoting popular proverbs about them. Luke, the author of the Gospel bearing his name, was called the "beloved physician."

Since God is obviously on the side of healing, our view is that medical technology is God's gift to humankind, enabling us to work toward curing disease and easing suffering, toward restoring our bodies to the health He desires for us all.

Modern medical science, then, is something we generally embrace as being morally good. We take antibiotics and undergo chemotherapy. We treat body, mind, and spirit as we seek health and well-being. We go to the doctor, *and* we spend time in prayer, believing that God will work through both to restore us to health. We find it hard to imagine that God would not expect us to do the same when facing infertility.

Clomid and pergonal, for example, are frequently prescribed fertility drugs that enhance the female body's reproductive capacities. There are chemical treatments for endometriosis and surgical procedures to open blocked fallopian tubes. There are drugs to augment sperm production and motility. These chemical and hormonal treatments merely serve to aid the body in carrying out its normal reproductive function.

In the early days of our treatment when both clomid and pergonal were prescribed by our specialist, Patricia thought no more of using them than she would taking aspirin for a headache. Ovulation-enhancing drugs pose no particular moral problems for those who understand medicine as an extension of God's healing hands.

Infertility Treatments and Their Moral Questions

Some infertility treatments, however, raise more difficult questions. With *in vitro* fertilization, for example, we are not merely curing disease; we are assisting in the creation of life.

Before undertaking any of these treatment options, talk with your doctor about which may be best suited to alleviating your particular problem. Ask questions so you can fully understand the procedure and its cost.

Check with your insurance company to see if you are covered for each recommended procedure. Some, like *in vitro* fertilization, are quite expensive and may not be covered under your medical plan.

Ask about the success rate. Realize that you may have to repeat the treatment several times, and that there is still a chance you might not become pregnant. Know that you will continue to ride the emotional roller coaster from cycle to cycle.

Talk openly and honestly with your spouse, your pastor, and your therapist. You and your spouse must agree on your chosen course of treatment. If you don't, the added stress could diminish your chances of successful conception and could lead to problems in your relationship.

If you have grieved over your situation and accepted the fact that you will not have a child in the usual way; if you have looked at adoption and decided that, for now at least, it isn't for you; if you and your spouse have agreed fully that you really do want to look into the alternatives; and if you have consulted with your specialist about which alternative methods might work best for you, then you are ready to move ahead and consider the moral questions.

Artificial Insemination

Artificial Insemination (AI) is a simple medical procedure. Semen obtained through masturbation is injected into the vagina, cervical canal, or uterus by means of a catheter. Usually warranted in cases of male sterility, AI is used to treat infertility stemming from impotence, genital malformation, low sperm count, low sperm motility, or where there is reason to believe that the male may pass on genetic disease or deformity.

Success rates vary and the process must normally be repeated several times before conception occurs. AI has a distinct advantage in that it is not nearly as expensive as some of the other methods.

There are two kinds of artificial insemination: Artificial Insemination by Husband (AIH), and Artificial Insemination by a Donor (AID).

Artificial insemination using the husband's sperm poses no serious moral problems. The husband and wife remain the primary participants and the medical procedure merely assists the procreative process.

Artificial Insemination by Donor (AID), however, introduces a third party, the sperm donor. AID means that the husband will not be the biological father of the child.

It takes a strong marriage to deal with AID. Since the husband must deal with feelings of failure over his inability to impregnate his wife, he may easily feel excluded from the process. His genetic heritage will not be carried on. The wife may have reservations about "carrying another man's child," and may feel a certain sense of guilt even though intercourse is not involved.

Because a third party is introduced into the procreative process, and because sperm must be obtained by masturbation, Roman Catholic moral theology considers AID to be adultery and the child illegitimate. Only children conceived through sexual intercourse between husband and wife are considered legitimate.

Protestant ethicists generally disagree. Since intercourse is not involved, AID is not considered adultery. Jesus taught that adultery was a matter of the heart (Matthew 5:27), not primarily the flesh. And there is no intercourse with anyone outside the marriage. With AID the procreative process still takes place in the context of a marriage where both parties want a child and are committed to parenting. It's therefore not usually considered any form of adultery.

AID does raise important emotional questions, though. Will you, the father, resent this child, knowing he or she isn't born of your sperm? Will you, the mother, feel this child has no real connection to your husband? Will either of you yearn to meet the man who fathered your child? Should you tell the child of his unusual conception?

These issues need to be dealt with openly before you proceed. If you have trouble dealing with them, then by all means get counseling. You are the ones who have to live with your decision—and take moral responsibility for it—whatever that decision may be.

You also will need to check the laws of your state. Most states now recognize the child conceived by AID as the legal offspring of the sperm recipient and her husband. But just as with adoption, it's best to make sure you have all the legal bases covered before you act.

In Vitro Fertilization

In vitro (literally, "in glass") fertilization is generally used to treat women with blocked or absent fallopian tubes, endometriosis, or men who have low sperm counts, and may include the use of donor semen and/or donor eggs. It is extremely expensive, usually upwards of $5,000 per attempt, and the procedure is rarely covered by insurance. Success rates are low, only 10–25 percent for each attempt.

Clinics carefully screen applicants. Generally the couple must be otherwise healthy and the woman between ages 25 and 30. They must be childless, have a stable marriage, have exhausted other suitable options, and demonstrate ability to pay all fees.

The procedure begins by stimulating ovum production, normally by administering clomid or pergonal. Estrogen levels are monitored through blood tests to determine when the eggs are ready, usually about 42 hours after the injection of fertility drugs. Ripened eggs are then removed by laparoscopy, a minor surgical procedure. Three to twelve eggs are collected.

The husband, or sperm donor, brings a fresh sample of semen to the clinic where it is "washed." Sperm washing separates sperm from seminal fluid by centrifuge. Sperm are then placed in a special solution that causes low-quality sperm to sink to the bottom while the more vital sperm rises to the top.

Sperm and ripened eggs are mixed in a laboratory dish and allowed to incubate for around 18 hours. Fertilized eggs are then removed from this solution and transferred to another where they are allowed to grow for approximately 38–40 hours. Three or four of the resulting embryos are transferred back to the woman through a catheter inserted into the cervical area where they are gently flushed into the uterus. She will lie very still for several hours to encourage implantation, then be dismissed to go home where further bed rest is recommended. Progesterone may be administered to facilitate implantation. After 10–14 days a pregnancy test is given to see whether implantation has occurred.

The Ethics Advisory Board

Though the first test-tube baby was born in England, American researchers also had been working on similar projects. In 1974, a professor at Vanderbilt University, Dr. Pierre Soupart, applied to the National Institutes of Health (NIH) for a grant to study the safety of *in vitro* fertilization. Recognizing the serious moral and legal questions that were sure to arise, the Department of Health, Education, and Welfare (now Health and Human Services), under the direction of Cabinet Secretary Joseph Califano and the Carter administration, appointed the Ethics Advisory Board (EAB) to look into all the legal, scientific, and moral questions surrounding *in vitro* fertilization.

From May 1978 until May 1979 the EAB held hearings interviewing infertile couples, theologians, legal scholars, feminist groups, right-to-life activists, researchers, and scientists. In their final report they concluded that, though there is danger of abuse in such procedures, these dangers were not sufficient to ban either *in vitro* research or the use of the procedure by physicians. The report reads in part:

> After much analysis and discussion regarding both scientific data and the moral status of the embryo . . . the embryo is entitled to profound respect, but this respect does not necessarily encompass the full legal and moral rights attributed to persons.[1]

The board made a key distinction between the embryo and the fetus. Whether *in vitro* fertilization is an option for you depends on whether you agree. Here you must face the question that has perplexed legal scholars, theologians, Supreme Court justices, and moralists for centuries: When does "human" life begin?

Roman Catholic moral theology holds the position that, because the unique genetic code of an individual is set the moment egg and sperm unite, human life begins at conception. The life of the embryo must therefore receive the same rights to protection afforded all other persons under our Constitution.

Furthermore, since only three or four embryos are inserted into the uterus, others must be either discarded or frozen for possible future use. Neither discarding nor freezing embryos is acceptable according to Roman Catholicism because the embryo is to be given all the rights and protections that should be given any fully mature person.

Protestant ethicists are divided on the question of when distinctively *human* life begins. Some agree with the Roman Catholic position that life begins at conception. Others generally agree with the EAB's distinction between the moral status of an embryo and that of a fetus which has developed to the point of viability (the point in time when the fetus is sufficiently developed to survive, with medical assistance, outside the womb). Those in agreement with the EAB recognize that while the embryo is *potentially* the beginning of a unique personal life, it is nonetheless *pre*-human, worthy of profound respect, but not equal to personal life.

In essence, this is the crucial distinction made by the Supreme Court in *Roe vs. Wade,* the 1973 decision legalizing abortion. The Court rejected the argument that the word *person* in the Fourteenth Amendment included the unborn. The justices wrote:

> We need not resolve the difficult question of when life begins. When those trained in the respective disciplines of medicine, philosophy and theology are unable to arrive at any consensus, the judiciary, at this point in the development of man's knowledge, is not in a position to speculate as to the answer (U.S. Supreme Court, *Roe v. Wade,* 410 U.S. 113, 1973).

Thus are we each left to make our own decisions and live out our own best convictions. However, as we stated earlier, when in doubt it's always best to go with the more conservative—in this case, Roman Catholic—position.

If, however, you decide *in vitro* fertilization is an option you would like to pursue, there are further ethical questions you must consider.

Transferring more than two or three embryos into the uterus, for example, increases the chances of multiple births, which may lead to undesirable complications. Therefore it's not uncommon to have embryos "left over" that may never be used, or to possibly face a crisis during pregnancy when one embryo may need to be aborted—a process called "selective" abortion—to save the other. Hence the question, "What is to be done with the extra embryos?"

There are currently three options. As mentioned earlier, embryos may be frozen for later use in the event early attempts fail. They also may be kept for research purposes, or they may be discarded. If you choose *in vitro* fertilization, you need to be actively involved in making the decision regarding the unused embryos.

Should you choose to have them frozen, know that there may be legal complications. An Australian couple, having frozen embryos for future use, was killed in a plane crash. The hospital had three choices: donate the embryos to another couple, to an approved research program, or dispose of them. In a more recent case a couple who had frozen some of their embryos was divorced. A bitter court battle followed over whether the father or mother would get "custody."

Such complicated matters illustrate the need for the contract with your fertility clinic or doctor to specify exactly what will happen to unused embryos. And though we do not like to think about such things, there is always the possibility of death or divorce. In a sense, you are making out a will, deciding what is to be done should you separate or one or both of you die.

Gamete IntraFallopian Transfer (GIFT)

Though GIFT is not helpful to women with blocked fallopian tubes, it is quite useful to couples where the male has inadequate sperm, or where the female has a cervix that makes it difficult for sperm to penetrate, suffers from endometriosis, or has a long history of otherwise unexplained infertility.

As with the *in vitro* procedure, ovulation-inducing drugs are administered to increase the number of ripening eggs. Semen is prepared by sperm "washing." Eggs are collected, examined for maturity, combined with sperm and injected through a laparoscopy incision into the end of the fallopian tubes.

Of all the methods we have considered, GIFT most closely mirrors the body's natural fertilization process. Fertilization takes place in the fallopian tube and the embryo descends into the uterus in the normal manner. The treatment is successful in about 60 percent of the cases.

GIFT also may be used by that small number of women who either lack ovaries or whose ovaries do not function. This process, sometimes known as "intrauterine adoption," involves the artificial insemination of a fertile "egg donor" with the semen from the infertile woman's husband. Prior to implantation in the egg donor's uterus, the fertilized egg is removed and transferred to the infertile wife who, barring other complications, is then able to carry the embryo to term.

Intrauterine adoption is new and not without its ethical problems. There is always a chance the egg donor may unintentionally become pregnant, at which time she will need to decide between carrying to term or abortion. Does the biological father have any rights or input into the egg donor's decision? Can the infertile couple be held legally responsible for the child should the donor proceed with the pregnancy? Could the infertile couple compel the egg donor to let them adopt the child?

These are questions our legal system is still grappling with, and there are as yet no definitive answers. But you should be aware of what might occur should you opt for this procedure and things not go as planned.

Conclusion

Fertility enhancing drugs, artificial insemination, *in vitro* fertilization, gamete intrafallopian transfer, and intrauterine adoption present alternatives for infertile couples who are able to take advantage of all modern medical science has to offer. As we have seen, each treatment is not appropriate for every infertile couple. And there are ethical issues to be considered before moving ahead with your particular options. Again, it is not our purpose to recommend any of these procedures. Our task has been merely to introduce the available options and raise the important ethical issues you need to consider before proceeding with any particular treatment.

Carefully and prayerfully consider the moral and legal ramifications confronting you. Go to the library and do your own research. Talk with your pastor and/or therapist. Ultimately you must make your own decisions, taking personal, moral, and legal responsibility for each.

No matter how well you do your homework, though, there may always be some doubt about whether you are doing the "right" thing. All you can do is put your trust in God. He knows we imperfect creatures will make mistakes as we bring our finite knowledge to the questions posed by our evolving technology. So make your decisions and move on with your life, content with the understanding that God knows we can do no more than live out our own best convictions.

THINGS TO DO

1. Check with your infertility specialist to determine which options might be suitable to your particular case.

2. Check with your insurance company to see whether these procedures are covered under your present policy.

3. If not, do you have the private financial resources to continue?

4. Carefully consider the moral questions involved in those treatment options available to you. Consult with your pastor. Read other texts that discuss the moral and legal problems in greater depths.

5. Be sure you make a decision you can live with, legally, morally, and spiritually. You alone bear responsibility for your decisions.

The moral and legal dilemmas of surrogate motherhood are at least complex, perhaps insurmountable.

10
Surrogate Motherhood

Jacob became angry with Rachel and said, "I can't take the place of God. He is the one who keeps you from having children."

Rachel said, "Here is my slave girl Bilhah; sleep with her so that she can have a child for me. In this way I can become a mother through her" (Genesis 30:2,3).

SURROGATE motherhood—as old as the Old Testament, as current as today's headlines. A process that opens a Pandora's box of legal, psychological, and ethical issues. In today's climate of rapidly advancing reproductive technology, these issues become increasingly complicated, and lawyers, courts, infertile couples, moralists, and civil libertarians are trying to find a way through the morass.

The method is simple—it's the rest of it that is so complex. As with *in vitro* fertilization, egg and sperm come from the couple who want the child, but the developing embryo is implanted in a woman who agrees to act as a surrogate mother.

The Old Testament brand of surrogacy differed greatly from today's practice, however. Women had few legal rights, and surrogacy was an accepted alternative to childlessness. In the Old Testament there was never any question as to whom the child belonged. The family patriarch had the final say. Children of surrogates were linked genetically to the ruling male, so there was never any question of the surrogate keeping the child as her own.

Today, with the advent of *in vitro* fertilization and with the ongoing struggle for women's reproductive rights and equal status under the law, the situation is radically different. *In vitro* fertilization makes it possible for the child to maintain the genetic link with both husband *and* wife. The surrogate offers her womb for a price and contracts to relinquish all rights to the child at birth. It sounds simple, but it doesn't always work out as intended.

In 1985 Mary Beth Whitehead agreed to be a surrogate mother for William and Elizabeth Stern. The Sterns agreed to pay Mrs. Whitehead $10,000 upon delivery. In return Mrs. Whitehead consented to give up all legal rights to the child. After delivery, Mrs. Whitehead wanted out of the contract, claiming she was too emotionally attached and was, after all, the "rightful" mother.

By 1987 the now-celebrated Whitehead case had made its way to the New Jersey Superior Court. In March of the same year the judge ruled that Mrs. Whitehead had no parental rights and ordered her to give up the child.

In a more recent case Mark and Crispina Calvert hired surrogate mother Anna Johnson to carry their biological child. When the baby was born Ms. Johnson, like Mrs. Whitehead, decided to keep the child. Santa Ana, California, Superior Court Judge Richard Parslow ruled in favor of the biological parents.

As we write this, Ms. Johnson vows to fight all the way to the Supreme Court to get "her" baby back. While this case has been settled, the ethical and legal questions will surely remain the subject of much debate.

According to Peter Volpe, author of *Test Tube Conception: A Blend of Love and Science*,[1] several hundred women in the U.S. have served as surrogate mothers. Only a few have contested parental rights.

We must emphasize that we are not recommending surrogacy as a viable alternative. However, any infertile couple researching their options will hear about surrogacy. Thus we feel responsible to address the issue here and to point out the practical, ethical, and moral dilemmas that must be considered.

Under certain circumstances, surrogacy might appear to be a good idea. There are many medical problems that make carrying a child to term extremely dangerous or impossible. Some women suffer from life-threatening kidney disorders, severe diabetes, or debilitating cardiac disease, or they have a history of repeated miscarriage. *In vitro* fertilization makes it possible for the infertile couple to maintain the genetic link.

Medical technology has made surrogacy a ready option—for those who can afford it. But is it morally defensible? Writes Volpe:

> Some ethicists object to surrogacy on the grounds that the practice constitutes economic exploitation of women . . . Detractors point out that it is as morally dis-

tasteful for a woman to bear a child for money as it is for a woman to ask money for sexual favors. Scientists themselves acknowledge that surrogacy is not a new medical advance but rather a commercial enterprise wherein motherhood is determined by contract . . . The novelty thus lies in treating babies like commodities.[2]

Some feminists and civil libertarians fear the profit motive might be strong enough to lure the poor into becoming something of a "breeder class" for those women who either cannot bear children, or who do not want to take time off for pregnancy and childbirth because it might interfere with their careers.

Yet those who become surrogates say they do so not for the money but out of a genuine desire to help the infertile couple. Generally the surrogate is in her mid-twenties, married, and has at least a high school or college degree. She enjoys pregnancy, the birth experience, and the extra attention she receives, according to P.J. Parker, author of "Motivation of Surrogate Mothers."[3]

Regardless of the surrogate's motives, however, she is much more than a human incubator. The health of the child in her womb depends on the surrogate's own psychological and physical health. What happens when the surrogate refuses to take care of herself?

For example, in 1977 a couple arranged a surrogate contract with a woman who appeared to be healthy and responsible. It turned out, however, that she was an alcoholic and gave birth to a child suffering from what is known as "fetal alcohol syndrome." In another case a surrogate gave birth to a child with microcephaly, a deformity resulting in mental retardation. Battles ensued over who had to take responsibility for the child.

The moral and legal dilemmas of surrogate motherhood are at least complex, perhaps insurmountable. Yet it is almost certain the practice will continue, if only because there is such widespread disagreement among ethicists and legal scholars about its legitimacy.

Surrogacy is banned under Roman Catholic moral theology for the same reason as *in vitro* fertilization. Yet even if we take the more accepting position on *in vitro* fertilization—that surrogacy does not constitute adultery because there's no sexual intercourse involved and the child will be the offspring of two parents who want him or her—serious moral problems remain.

Though the basic process is the same in surrogacy as with Artificial Insemination by a Donor (AID), there is one *crucial* distinction. With AID the donor is not identified. Surrogacy introduces a fully adult third party, well known by and under contract to the infertile couple. While most states have laws designating AID children to be the legal offspring of the biological father, current laws on surrogacy are at best ambiguous, at worst nonexistent. Hence the very real possibility for custody fights like those we have described above.

Surrogates must build an emotional wall between themselves and the child in their wombs. We simply do not know whether this type of psychological detachment will in the long run be damaging to the child. What we do know is that surrogates, after delivery, often experience feelings of depression, profound loss, guilt, and rejection.[4]

Even when the surrogate is motivated by compassionate concern for the infertile couple, the deliberate conception of a child out of wedlock is not something to be taken lightly. "Women," writes D. Garth Jones, referring to the surrogate, "are not simply machines able to develop prod-ucts without serious attachment to the product itself."[5]

We no longer live in the patriarchal world of the Old Testament. Besides, just because examples of surrogacy can be found in Scripture does not mean we should approve the practice without critical reflection.

Modern surrogacy may at best be an example of com-passion carried too far. At worst it may be another way poor women can sell—or, more precisely, rent—their bodies for purely monetary reasons.

The surrogate acts outside any context of loving com-mitment to the child's father or mother. Surrogate mothers are reduced to the mere biological reproduction of a child for someone else. Hence the argument that the practice is so demeaning to women that it should be banned outright. Still others argue that those who choose to become sur-rogate mothers should have the right to do so, since their bodies are their own.

Conclusion

Surrogacy is one of those unfolding areas of moral and legal affairs where carefully crafted legislation based on hard thinking about the myriad of ethical questions is needed to protect the rights and concern of everyone involved.

Before you consider surrogacy you need to hire an attorney who is familiar with the laws governing your state. Know that your life will be inextricably bound with that of the surrogate mother, since she knows you and will have no trouble finding you. Ask yourself whether you would be willing to grant the surrogate visitation rights should she wish to remain in contact. All these decisions should be carefully spelled out in your contract—a contract that could be disputed even after the child is born, plunging you into a bitter, expensive court battle.

There is one final question that ranks among the most important of all: Are you willing to accept the child should it be born mentally or physically impaired? If not, then we do not believe you should attempt the surrogate option. A child is a gift of God, however it comes to us—not a television you can take back if you decide you don't like the quality of the picture. Surrogacy, unlike adoption, does not offer us the option of deciding beforehand whether we have what it takes to parent the special-needs child. Remember, in surrogacy the child is a product of *your* genes, not those of the surrogate.

Most of the time surrogacy contracts work out as planned. Surrogacy can work. But as we have seen, there are many pitfalls to be avoided, many opportunities for something to go wrong. You risk much when entering a surrogacy agreement: substantial amounts of money, the possibility of protracted litigation, a child psychologically or physically impaired due to a surrogate not taking proper care of herself, the possible economic exploitation of the surrogate who may be motivated by financial need, even the chance of losing your biological child.

Whether all these risks outweigh the possible gain, and whether, risks aside, the option of surrogacy falls within your moral and religious worldview, is something you must prayerfully decide.

THINGS TO DO

1. If you are interested in pursuing the possibility of finding a surrogate mother, the first and most important thing you must do is find a reputable attorney skilled in the laws governing surrogacy in your area.

2. Thoroughly review all the moral arguments and possible legal difficulties surrounding this issue. Prayerfully decide whether you can take the legal risks, moral responsibilities, and financial burdens surrogacy will impose on you as a couple.

3. Understand that you are dealing in an area where the laws are still changing. This means you must be emotionally and spiritually prepared for currently unforeseeable problems and setbacks in the process.

Epilogue

IN THESE pages Patricia and I have shared our personal struggles, something of our faith journeys, and the fruits of our learning and research into the complex and painful subject of infertility. We realize your journey through these trying circumstances will be uniquely yours. Yet if you have been honest with yourself you probably have found something of your own feelings, thoughts, and even prayers in these pages. Given more time, chances are you will find even more of your own ups and downs recorded here when you reread selected passages.

As we leave you to follow your own path, we encourage you to do just that—go back and read portions of this book again and again as they apply to your own faith journey. We have written in hopes that through our sharing we might be your fellow traveler.

Unfortunately, neither the human spirit nor the body can heal as quickly as one can read through a short book. We all know life is not that simple.

What we do know is that your struggle with infertility will come to a resolution. You will conceive and bear a child, or you will adopt, or you will remain childless. The grief, the emotional highs and lows, the marital stress, doctors visits, tests, and treatments will eventually cease. However this particular chapter in your life ends, know that you can, if you choose to do your own spiritual and emotional work, move successfully into the next stage of your lives together.

We hope, as we're sure you do, that your story ends happily. But we also know that it will not for everyone. Our lives are not fairy tales. We live in a very real world where dreams don't always come true. Our lives sometimes do not turn out quite as we had planned.

The only certainty any of us really have is the assurance that God's magnificent grace will never abandon us, and that this amazing grace will be sufficient for all our needs.

Go with God.

Alan G. Trent
Patricia Hatfield Trent

Notes

Chapter 1

1. Marilyn Larkin, "When the Body Says No," *Health* (June 1985), p. 54.
2. Robert H. Blank, "Making Babies: The State of the Art," *Futurist* (February 1985), p. 17.
3. Blank, p. 17.
4. Larkin, p. 56.
5. Larkin, p. 54.
6. Larkin, p. 54.

Chapter 2

1. Lynda R. Stephenson, *Give Us A Child: Coping With the Personal Crisis of Infertility* (San Francisco: Harper and Row, 1987), p. 17.

Chapter 3

1. Barbara Eck Menning, *Infertility: A Guide for Childless Couples* (Englewood Cliffs: Prentice Hall, Inc., 1977), p. 109.

Chapter 4

1. Lori B. Andrews, *New Conceptions: A Consumer's Guide to the Newest Infertility Treatments* (New York: St. Martin's Press, 1984), pp. 99–100.

Chapter 9

1. Ethics Advisory Board. Two Volumes: *Report* and *Conclusions* (Washington, D.C.: Department of Health, Education and Welfare, May 4, 1979).

Chapter 10

1. Peter Volpe, *Test-Tube Conception: A Blend of Love and Science* (Macon: Mercer University Press, 1987), pp. 63–9.
2. Volpe, p. 64.
3. Cited by Volpe, p. 65.
4. P.J. Parker, "Motivation of Surrogate Mothers: Initial Findings," *American Journal of Psychiatry* (1983) 40:117–8.
5. D. Garth Jones, *Brave New People: Ethical Issues at the Commencement of Life* (Grand Rapids: William B. Eerdmans, 1985), pp. 179–80.

Real Help
for Real Hurts